MW01593841

HIGH HEELS IN LOW PLACES

Meet everyday women with miraculous testimonies who will ignite your Faith & Hope to fight Breast Cancer.

A Compilation Presented By
Tamekia Hunter Ross

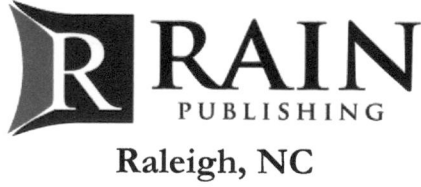

RAIN
PUBLISHING

Raleigh, NC

Rain Publishing
www.rainpublishing.com

Crafted To Motivate, LLC
www.craftedtomotivate.com

Book Cover Design – John Linzie
Edited By Dr. Damion Lewis

High Heels In Low Places/ Tamekia Hunter Ross – 1st ed.
ISBN 979-8-9855005-5-4

Library of Congress Control Number: 2022912199

Foreword

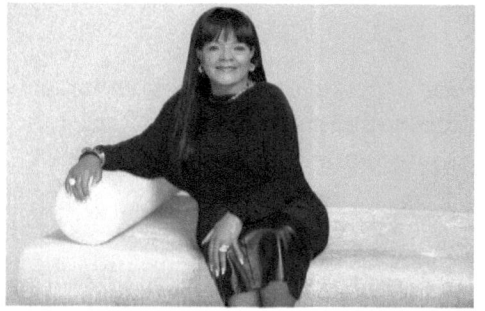

Our God is a faithful God, even in difficult times that appear to be seemingly hopeless. As women striving to stand on God's principles, we know that it is only by His grace & mercy; and the faith we have in Christ that strengthens us to always keep our hope in Him. His miracle working power equips us with the strength to have a victorious mindset regardless of the trials we face.

This book is a beautiful compilation of stories of women who have decided to walk powerfully through their bout with cancer and have declared that they will walk with their hope solely in Christ Jesus. Their stories will move your spirit to come into total faith and be fully persuaded that God is in control. Some of them are currently walking through the fire, some have already made it through, but every single one of them made a decision to walk through it in faith.

Thus, if you are looking to be inspired, if you are yearning for hope in a hopeless situation, and if you are searching for an earthly example of God's faithfulness; you will find it in this compilation of these women's faith challenging experiences. May each of their shared stories quicken your spirit to move from faith to faith to more faith; and may they bless your spirit as it has mine.

I would also like to encourage every contributor who shared their experience in this volume to keep holding on to faith knowing that your story is going to be a light to others who will walk this same path.

Love, Because of Calvary,

Pastor Shirley Caesar

Dedication

On behalf of all of the "High Heels In Low Places" BREASTies, we dedicate this book to:

Thrivers who are currently active in any type of treatment whether it be chemotherapy, radiation, preparing or recovering from surgery. Remember, "I can do ALL things through Christ who strengthens me" (Philippians 4:13)

Metavivors who were diagnosed with Stage IV as a result of the breast cancer returning or spreading to other parts of the body. We are constantly lifting you in prayer and are always here to support you and cheer you on from the side lines and will get in the "trenches" with you. No matter what science, doctors or statistics say, Walk by Faith trusting and believing God for His Word "This sickness is not unto death, but for the glory of God, so that the Son of God may be glorified by it." (John 11:4)

Survivors who fought, conquered and won! We understand that life will never be the same and survivors have to adjust to a new normal of the many ways breast cancer affected them mentally, emotionally, financially and physically. Take back everything the devil stole from you and as you continue living life in your new normal, take everything you learned and become a healthier you so you never have to deal with it again. Eat and exercise and stay away from harmful toxins and chemicals as if your life depended on it. Now that you have survived and overcome, let not your journey be in vain. Educate your family, friends and community and support those still in the fight. Your "giving back" can not only change a life but save a life. We celebrate with you and we say "thanks be to God, who gives us the victory through Jesus Christ." (1 Corinthians 15:57),

The Taken who received their healing on the other side, in heaven. Our heart breaks and aches every time we hear of the death of a BREASTie to breast cancer. As Christians, believers and women of Faith, the bible teaches us that we not only live in Faith but we also die in Faith. Breast Cancer never wins and we never lose to Breast Cancer. The Taken not only received their ultimate healing but they also received the most ultimate reward anyone can have when we have served our purpose in the earth. "To be absent from the body is to be present with the Lord". (2 Corinthians 5:8)

"O Lord my God, I cried to You and You have healed me"
Psalm 30:2

Acknowledgment

To my creator, who gave His only begotten son, Jesus Christ, not only for our sins but also for our sickness and diseases. Lord, I thank you for giving me the courage and strength to live in Faith and walk-in Faith trusting you for the provision of the vision. You get ALL the Glory through my life. It's never about me, but all about Jesus.

To my husband, **Arnteyus** "Jay." Thank you for all the sacrifices you make in being my primary caregiver and ensuring I get to Atlanta every three weeks for treatment and appointments. Thank you for keeping your promise to God to love me "in sickness and in health". I love you with all my heart and appreciate all that you do. To my sons, **Cameron** and **Caleb**. I hope I have lived and continue to live a life as an example that no matter what life may bring us, we can do ALL things through Christ who strengthens us. Never let any sickness, disease, or anyone stop you from being all that God created you to be. No one in this world will ever love you more and believe in you more than your mom. I love you sons! To my mom, **Maggie Sumter Hunter,** and my three older brothers: **Rodney**, **Marvin,** and **Sean**. Family, I can't even fathom how my diagnosis affected you all after losing dad to cancer. Despite what we all went through emotionally with dad, especially mom, you all have been there. Mom, you have always been my biggest cheerleader on the sidelines, alongside my husband Jay. We thank you all for the love, support, and prayers. To **Angelia "Angie" Gibson Neal**, my cousin by marriage who became my "SisterCousin" and bestie. You have not only been there for me but supported my entire family. You are the true representation of family and a real, genuine friend and "sistah" that I can ALWAYS trust and depend on. You are truly a woman of "noble character" (Proverbs 31) and I thank God for you daily. I love you with all my heart chic!

To my **BREASTies**, Thank you for trusting the God inside of me to write, birth and carry out the vision so together we can make a difference regarding breast cancer. We are stronger together and I thank God daily for each of you. I love you with all of my heart and there is nothing you can do about it!

A special "thank you" to the best Oncologist and care team on this side of Heaven, Dr. John E. McKnight and the Cancer Treatment Centers of Newnan along with the friendliest and most caring Patient Relationship Manager, Erin DeSart.

Introduction

We all at some point in our life used to be just like our daughters and nieces who would play and walk around in their mother's shoes and play dress-up. Some call it playing grown up. Most every woman we know has a love for heels. Our closets are packed to capacity with all of our heels and favorite shoes. We take much preparation and pride in presenting ourselves and our appearance to the world. As good as we look, and as appealing as the right pair of heels sets off that perfect outfit, in one out of every ten thousand pairs of heels is a woman who has, who is, or who will experience a low place in her life caused by a breast cancer diagnosis. It is important to note that, "African American women have a 31% breast cancer mortality rate–the highest of any U.S. racial or ethnic group. Among women younger than 45, breast cancer incidence is higher among African American women than White women." (BCPP)

Just like every woman, as little girls, we all dreamed of a life full of love, laughter, and happy endings. We all have experienced love and laughter in our life but some of us have also experienced some of life's experiences that deferred our happy endings caused by breast cancer. As breast cancer survivors, thrivers, and "metavivors", we all have had a low place in our life we refused to acknowledge or talk about it to anyone. But most importantly, we refuse to release it to God and fully trust Him. Instead, we find ourselves in emotional and spiritual warfare with our minds because of that one question we never seemed to find the answer to, "God why me?" No matter how fabulous we present ourselves to others from head to toe, all of us are carrying some weight that we need to release regarding our breast cancer diagnosis and journey.

Some of us are known for our stylish stilettos, kitten heels, sling-backs, wedges, or pumps. We all have that one favorite pair of heels we enjoy wearing whenever we can. No matter the event, the occasion, the style or attire, after being in a pair of heels for a long period of time, our feet begin to get tired and hurt and require relief. There is nothing like being able to wear a nice pair of heels that are comfortable and cause no pain. God desires the same from us when it comes to our bodies and our physical healing. He desires that we live a life of abundance. "Beloved, I wish above all things that thou mayest prosper and be in health, even as thy soul prospereth." (3 John 2)

High Heels in Low Places offers hope and encouragement to breast cancer survivors, thrivers, and metavivors to cry out to God to not only heal you from your physical scars but also from all of the emotions and low places your breast cancer journey took you through. Psalms 30:2 "Lord my God, I called to you for help, and you healed me."

No matter your age, religion, social background, or years of remission, when we begin to really cry out to God to help us with all the hurt and disappointment caused by breast cancer, we can really begin our true and real healing not only physically, but emotionally and mentally.

We all desire to be greater individuals and to make a difference, not only in this world but in someone else's life. But how can we be effective and make a difference when no one wants to be open, honest, real, and transparent about the low places we experienced from breast cancer. These journeys were not for us, but to help someone else along the way. We found and discovered how strong we really are.

So many of us begin each new day with our usual routine of putting all of our energy and thoughts into our outer appearance presentation. As women, we take much pride in how we look and how we carry ourselves. Besides, appearance is everything...right? Some of us go to the extremes of paying attention to every detail of our attire. From hair to makeup, makeup to undergarments, undergarments to accessories, and from accessories to our attire. Then to set it all off and sum it up, we put on the perfect pair of heels to seal the deal. What is so funny about us as women, if the shoes don't work with our attire, we will change our attire before we will change our heels if we feel like something is not working. Yes, we really do that. That is why we are always late. HAHA. So why can't we take that same attitude to live healthy lives to prevent and decrease the breast cancer rate, especially among African American women including reoccurrence? As we pay closer attention to the details on our inside, we can have a better effect on how we handle what is on the outside.

Why is it that we take so much time and give so much detail to our outer appearance, but we spend very little time with what is going on inside of us? Why are we afraid to discuss and reveal those low places in our lives from our breast cancer journeys? We would rather dress up our low places with an expensive pair of designer shoes, to make us feel good for a moment. But then when we step out of our heels, we step back into those low places where we hide and dress up. So many of us need to admit how breast cancer has hurt us, changed us, and affected us so we can cry out to God and allow Him to not only heal us from the disease and physical scars but for all the emotions tied in with it as well. One thing about a good pair of heels, especially our favorite pair, if we don't take care of them, the places our heels tread whether it be dirt, gravel, pavement, water, or grass, can cause not only wear and tear but physical damage to our heels as well. We walk by faith and not by the diagnosis. No matter where our heels take us or the type of ground they may sink into, we can't stay there. Just like heels, we must dust ourselves off, remove all the dirt, mud, grass, and water and keep going. And keep fighting through the journey. Life does not stop. Everyone will not always be kind, considerate of your diagnosis, supportive, or concerned. But we fight and keep fighting as if our lives depend on it, no matter who is in the ring with us or who is on the outside of the ring cheering us on. We have to be our biggest advocates and our biggest fans. We can't expect anyone to admire our heels if we don't first admire them. Love and support yourselves more than you can ever expect, want or ask anyone else to.

Every day someone is diagnosed with breast cancer. Every day someone dies from breast cancer. But more of the women diagnosed with breast cancer and dying from breast cancer, are women of color who look more like me. So what can we do to decrease the numbers and the statistics? Glad you asked. We got to have faith! No matter what the doctor says, no matter what statistics say, and no matter what happens to other women and men diagnosed with breast cancer. We must have faith and walk by faith. Faith is the substance of things hoped for, the evidence of things not seen. If we have faith the size of a mustard seed, God can do the impossible.

I personally had to first learn to speak from faith and not from emotions. Now, I can live and lead by example to my BREASTies. Life and death are in the power of our tongues and as long as we believe, have faith, and give God back His word that He is able to perform just what He promises.

No matter how many repeats of scans, chemotherapy, radiation, surgeries, or appointments we have to go through–keep the faith. Even when we get tired, keep the faith! As life continues to go on around us, not compromising nor sympathizing with our diagnosis and journey, keep the faith!

The purpose of this book is to activate your faith through our transparency and real-life stories regarding our breast cancer diagnosis and journey. It is our hope that our openness and realness not only activate your faith but educate and inform you of those red flags and warning signs so many people miss in the beginning.

The co-authors (aka "BREASTies") come from different socioeconomic backgrounds, diverse childhoods, careers, ages, household compositions, and overall, different breast cancer experiences. Some of us may have had the same stage and same type of diagnosis (Triple Negative, HER2 Negative, HER2 Positive, etc). But because our bodies are different, our stories and journeys are different. They were asked to write and express their journeys in a format that will give you hope and activate your faith like never before. Some of the BREASTies shared their journeys of overcoming adversity, family, and job-related issues affected by their diagnosis. While others provided information and advice on warning signs, prevention, and better self-care. Overall, all BREASTies were intentional about ensuring you receive a message and resume life with faith, hope, and love.

You may have received this book from someone who loves you as being a thriver, metavivor or survivor. Or, maybe it was a book that you decided to read out of curiosity or to support our purpose and cause. Regardless of how you encountered **High Heels In Low Places**, it was placed in your life for a purpose. See, what you hold in your hand is a piece of African American history. An instant collectable item that can be shared with generations to come. No matter the moment in time, this book will serve as a tool to guide you and future generations on the prevention, awareness, and victories regarding breast cancer.

High Heels In Low Places is also our call to action to prove that we not only talk by faith but we walk by faith. We not only walk by faith, but we are stronger together in faith. The stronger we become in our faith, the more we will see fewer women of color diagnosed and affected by breast cancer. The Bible tells us that "the people perish for a lack of knowledge (wisdom)". As a people, we no longer have an excuse to be defeated by breast cancer. **High Heels in Low Places** is giving you a reason to not only fight in faith but keep the faith. Through our faith, we can close the health disparity gap among African American women and continue to overcome breast cancer by the blood of the lamb and through the words of our testimonies. (Revelation 12:11) Science and doctors may not have a cure for metastatic breast cancer. but our faith tells us that our God is bigger than cancer and Jesus is the cure! It is our prayer through our journeys and testimonies that someone gets to know Jesus while someone else just remembers who He is and the price Jesus has already paid on the cross, not only for our sins but also for sickness and diseases. As we continue to educate, bring awareness, and advocate, we pray and hope that you heal from what low place you may be in, whether it be breast cancer, finances, martial, etc. Whatever it is, it's time to heal thyself!

Let's begin exploring the lives and journeys of bold and courageous women of color who share their truths about the low places through their breast cancer journey. Discover the truth of our low places, but remember the victories we have won by being healed emotionally, mentally, and physically. So go and grab some snacks, and that favorite beverage, and find a quiet place that will allow you to read this book without many distractions. You are about to take a journey into the "shoe closets" of a special group of survivors and thrivers as we share our journeys, our low places, but most of all our places of healing and wholeness after being broken. I hope you find laughter, tears of joy, encouragement, hope, and faith. Let's begin to heal ourselves!

"*Women & Heels*
Tell me about your heels
&
I'll tell you who you are . . ."

-Author Unknown

Table of Contents

"Life is like a blank book, you write your own story not others."
– Zihan Zheng

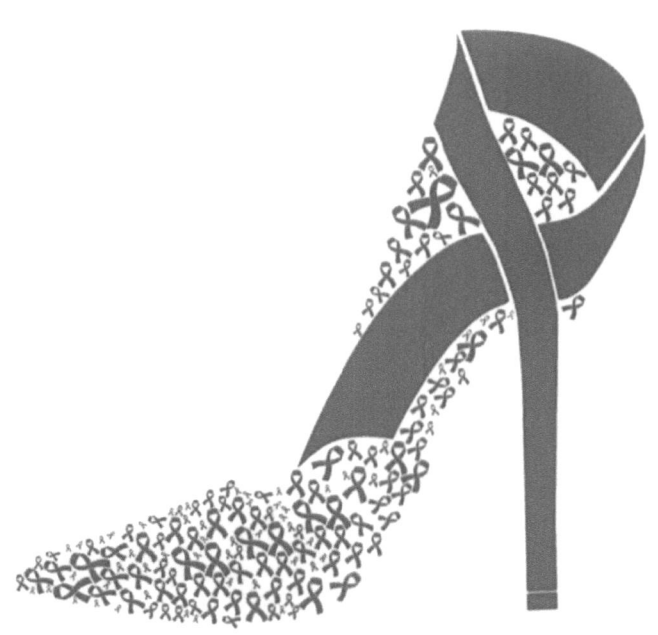

HIGH HEELS IN LOW PLACES

The collected memoirs of this text are presented with much of their original, vernacular language. As these are the memoirs of heroines who have and continue to defy impossible odds, their stories have been offered in this manner.

Cancer Broke My Heart..But It Did Not Break My Faith
Tamekia Hunter Ross

My journey and heartbreak from cancer started in 2011, years before my first diagnosis of breast cancer. In 2011, my dad was diagnosed with prostate cancer while I was living in Atlanta, rebuilding my life from my second marriage. Now let me give you some history concerning my dad and me. To really know me is to know that I am daddy's girl. I am the youngest and only girl of four siblings, and my dad has always been the first man I ever loved and loved with my whole heart. I was spoiled, very spoiled, and loved by my dad until he took his last breath at 10:13 AM Thursday, August 14, 2014. I don't know what it is like to be without, what it is like to struggle, and what it is like to do things on my own. Because for my entire life, I always had my dad to do all of that for me.

I remember I was working at a big firm in downtown Atlanta the day I learned that my dad was diagnosed with prostate cancer. It literally shattered my heart into a thousand pieces. Within less than 24 hours of learning about my dad's diagnosis, the firm I was working for at that time announced to the staff that they were closing due to financial reasons. As much as I wanted to be disappointed and upset, I could not. I saw that as God's way of telling me to "go home and help your mom take care of your dad". So what I thought was something devastating, becoming unemployed, became a blessing in disguise. As soon as the firm closed, I relocated back to Sumter, South Carolina, and moved in with my parents.

By the time I relocated to Sumter, my dad was recovering from his surgery and just about to start radiation. I must admit, this diagnosis may have slowed my dad down but he did not miss a beat of continuing to live his life. I believe this was more of a transition and adjustment for me than it was for my dad. Here I was, 38 years old and back at home since graduating from high school and living with my parents as a single mom with two boys. I had not lived in Sumter since I graduated from college in 1996. As excited as I was to be back at home, near and close to my dad, when reality really set in, I kept asking myself: "what was I thinking?" I have become so accustomed to certain environments, and people, that it felt like moving from the city to the country.

Well, things went well and my dad kicked cancer's butt even after being a severe diabetic since he was a child. It did not take long before my dad was back to doing everything he was doing before being diagnosed with prostate cancer.

But low and behold, our family was faced with cancer again in 2013 and this time it came back like a vengeance, terrorizing our family and leaving us with broken hearts over, and over, and over, again. In 2013, my dad started having issues in his body that we could not explain, nor could doctors determine what was causing it. The first issue was a persistent dry cough that was so bad that you thought my dad would cough up a lung. My dad was a smoker all of his life, so they kept linking the cough with his smoking. A couple of months later my dad started having very sharp pains in his stomach. Pains so bad that there were numerous days we would find him in a fetal position on a floor because the pain was unbearable. It broke my heart to see my dad in so much pain. I felt helpless.

As life continued, and my dad continued incurring symptoms, discomfort, and pain without any answers from doctors, life took a very tragic twist for us. For weeks and months, my dad was in and out of the doctor's offices, the ER, and the hospital, but yet no one could tell us what was wrong with my dad. While trying to figure out what was going on with my dad, our family went through the unimaginable.

Our next heartbreak came on Labor Day weekend. My dad was the caregiver and guardian of one of his older brothers, also my uncle. We all went to our family church together and you will always find my uncle being the first to arrive every Sunday morning at church for Sunday school. This particular first Sunday, Labor Day weekend, my dad arrived at church and noticed that his brother's (my uncle) car was not there, and he is always the first to arrive on Sunday mornings. As my dad went into the church for Sunday school, he also noticed my uncle was not inside. He just assumed he was running late, which was unusual for him because he would at least call my dad to let him know he was not coming.

By the time Sunday school was over and church services were ready to begin, my dad became worried because not only did my uncle never appear, he never called my dad. My dad stepped outside to call his brother, but he did not answer, nor return any of my dad's calls. At this point, my dad knew something was wrong. He left the church and met his sister (my aunt) at his brother's house, which was located only a mile from the church. I remember my mom calling me to let me know my dad was leaving the church to go and check on his brother and she wanted me to check on my dad. So instead of waiting to hear from my dad or mom, I left the gym that morning and picked up my baby boy from my aunt, and went straight to my uncle's house to see what was going on. When I arrived at my uncle's house, I saw my dad and my aunt's car in the yard. I got out of my car and walked into my uncle's house and saw both my dad and his sister, one on each side of the chair that my uncle was kneeling in as if he was praying. But unfortunately, he was not praying. My dad found his brother, my uncle, dead in his house. My uncle died from COPD as a result of lung cancer.

When I say that Labor Day weekend was a holiday I would never forget. That would be an understatement. That day, and the loss of my uncle, was just the beginning of our family nightmare and heartbreak from cancer. That was the first death my dad's immediate family had experienced in years, decades. It was the first time I had ever seen that side of my dad or seen him cry so uncontrollably that it broke me to my knees. I am a daddy's girl so when my dad cried and hurt, so did I.

We went through the process of planning and preparing for my uncle's funeral. His death brought family members, and friends from the community I had not seen in years. It also brought our family closer because it's been a long time, years, and decades since we had to experience death. As we prepared and celebrated the life of my uncle, we tried our best to go on with our new normal of living life without him. Just when we thought the pain and grieving were getting better, less than 60 days from losing my uncle, we lost yet another uncle and brother to cancer. This time throat cancer.

By this time, I was in so much shock and disbelief that we were going through this again, that I was very numb and did not even know how to grieve. My emotions were all over the place and my heart was heavy, very heavy. So here we go again, planning and preparing to celebrate the life of yet another one of my dad's brothers.

As a family, we made it through another heartbreak of death and cancer. It was not easy, but we coped the best we knew how to. Even while dealing with the unexpected and sudden deaths, we were still faced with my dad's own medical issues and symptoms that no one could find a diagnosis for. My dad continued to be in pain while grieving the loss of his two older brothers. He continued to be in and out of doctor's appointments, the ER, and the hospital from all the pain he was experiencing, and still, no one was able to tell us anything.

To get my mind off things, I started planning my 40th birthday for January 2014. I took all of my time and energy and started planning something different and unique to help me cope with my grief and heartbreaks. My 40th birthday weekend was a weekend to remember, and it brought me so much joy and happiness, despite all of my sorrow and grief. I remember when I came back home that weekend, after being in Columbia celebrating with friends. I remember my dad calling me outside to sit with him and we talked. I was good that weekend, so I was uncertain as to what I had done wrong. Normally, if my dad is pulling me to the side to that extent, I either did something wrong or he was preparing me for something.

Needless to say, I did nothing wrong, but at that point and time, I did not realize he was preparing me for something. We continued to talk and he asked me about my birthday weekend, the dinner, the party, etc. Then he said something that caught me off guard, "I noticed you stopped going to church and have not been in months". If you could see the look on my face, I was like a deer in headlights. I did not see that coming! My dad just reminded me how they raised us to be in church on Sunday mornings unless we were sick and he reminded me that as a young single mom and everything that we just went through as a family, I needed to be in someone's church on Sunday mornings.

Being the daddy's girl that I am, I took everything my dad said to me to heart. I started visiting different churches in the area and could not just seem to find what I felt was best for me and my boys. Then I remembered a childhood classmate of mine since the 6th grade who was constantly inviting me to come to his church which was less than a half-mile from our house. The following weekend after my dad and I had this conversation, I immediately started going to a church down the street from my house. Little did I know that was the best advice and decision I could have made, not realizing it was needed to prepare me for what was ahead.

As I was enjoying my new church and new church family, my dad continued to struggle with his medical issues, and here we were, a year later, and no one could still tell us what was going on with my dad. It was May 2014, my dad was in so much pain we called 9-1-1. And he was later transported and admitted to the hospital again. This time, the doctor on call, who was treating my dad, noticed that there was fluid on my dad's lungs and stomach. He immediately scheduled a biopsy to have the fluid drained and sent to Charleston to find answers to my dad's problem.

Memorial weekend is never the same for me anymore because that Friday of memorial weekend 2014, we received the results of my dad's biopsy, Stage IV Mesothelioma Cancer. What? Why? How? Numerous other questions began to go through my mind as uncontrollable tears flowed from my face. I became very angry for many reasons as questions continue to linger in my head. I felt like someone was responsible and I wanted to blame someone for this.

My dad immediately began chemotherapy right after the diagnosis. Shortly after the first chemotherapy, once again, cancer broke our hearts and my dad's oldest brother passed away in June of 2014. By now, you can't even imagine how we are feeling and what we are going through as a family. A part of me wanted to scream, while another part of me wanted to cry while another part of me wanted to have a nervous breakdown. But as a daddy's girl, I had to be strong for my dad. I was just a niece, so I can't begin to fathom how my dad was feeling and what he was going through in his mind to lose three brothers, back-to-back, to Cancer, and then be diagnosed himself with Cancer.

Very weak, fragile, and frail my dad once again buried a third brother while himself going through a cancer battle. Right after burying his brother, my dad completed his second round of chemotherapy. After this second round, things took a turn for the worse for my dad. He became weaker and lost so much weight that it was just as if his skin was hanging off his bones. With my dad being a diabetic all of his life since he was a child and taking insulin three to four times a day, along with the harshest chemotherapy, his body could not take it. He stayed in and out of the hospital and was constantly sick after that second round of chemotherapy.

His last time in the hospital was during my youngest son's birthday. I remembered taking cake and ice cream and celebrating with my dad in the hospital. My dad was very quiet during this visit, which is not like him, especially when my boys are around. I just assumed he was tired from all of the meds. It was not until a couple of weeks later, the weekend of our family reunion, that my mom informed us that when my dad was released from the hospital they told my parents there was nothing else they could do for my dad and they were sending him home on hospice care. When I say I felt like someone punched me in my gut and in my chest and all I remember doing was running out of the house screaming and yelling to the top of my lungs. Again, Why? How? When? Along with questions that I needed answers for. Why my dad? I remember crying for hours and could not sleep that Sunday night. I was devastated and heartbroken and as numb as numb could be. The next day when I went to work I was in so much disbelief, emotional, and heartbroken I could not even focus and concentrate on my work and asked to take a leave of absence. My employer could see the pain and hurt in my eyes that they even allowed me to leave work early that Monday. I went straight home, changed clothes, and just laid in the bed next to my dad and was determined to do that every day that God allowed him to be here with me.

Less than 24 hours after taking my leave from work, the hospice nurse came in that Tuesday to check on my dad. After checking on my dad she came into the kitchen and informed my mom and me that my dad had started transitioning and he will take his final flight by the weekend. I'm like what? Wait? What are you talking about? Hell, I am still trying to process the fact that they said there is nothing else they can do for my dad and now you are telling me that my dad is literally dying in front of my eyes?

I remember my pastor being the first person I called because I was literally about to lose it, and I felt my faith shaking. I wanted to question God.

It was at this very moment that I realized that the talk my dad had with me about church was preparing me for this very moment that I thought I would not have to face anytime soon. We had just lost three brothers, three uncles, and now my dad. Heartbroken is not even a strong enough word to describe that pain. I began to start replaying sermons, reading scriptures, and listening to gospel songs to give me the strength I needed to get through this heartbreak.

Family and closest friends began to come to our home that Tuesday afternoon to see my dad while he was still alert, even though he was not talking. Every chance I got, I lay in bed next to my dad listening to his heartbeat and telling him how much I loved him.

My youngest brother was in Texas, while my middle brother was in Virginia, and my oldest brother was in Jacksonville. My oldest brother literally just left Sumter that Sunday evening after the first devastating news, and by the time he got to Jacksonville, he was coming back to Sumter. And he was there with my mom and me at our family home as my dad continued his transition.

I will never forget that Wednesday night my mom, oldest brother, and I experienced things we had never experienced before. We sat and watched, heard, and observed my dad go through his final phases of life on earth. From the death rattle to the lifeless moments. That night was the longest and hardest night of my life. It took my mom and brother peeling me from his bedside to leave my dad even just for a second. As I was preparing to take my son to daycare, a hospice nurse came in and informed us that my dad was in his final stages and the next time he opened his eyes would be his last time of being able to hear us before he took his last breath. By this time, I didn't even want to leave to take my son to daycare, but I did. I know I drove about 100mph trying to get there and back to be there with my dad.

When I returned, less than 15 minutes had passed, and everyone was sitting in the kitchen. I went straight into the bedroom and the moment I walked in and lay in the bed next to my dad, he opened his eyes. I yelled out and my mom, oldest brother and the nurse immediately came. We all took turns talking to my dad while stroking his hair, rubbing his head and his hands just reminding him how much we love him and ensuring him we were going to be okay. After five minutes, my dad closed his eyes and continued to take long deep breaths. The hospice nurse kept telling us he is still holding on and waiting for you all to let him go. We called both my brothers that were not there and held the phone to his ear while they talked to dad. Ten minutes later he was still taking the long deep breaths. So we called my Godfather, my dad's best friend of 60 years whom he talked to every morning. My Godfather talked to my dad just like he did every morning and even sang my dad's favorite song. Ten minutes, now almost thirty minutes and my dad was still taking shallow breaths. The nurse asked us if there was anyone else we needed to call. My mom told the nurse that there was no one left to call and that I needed to let my dad go and that I was the reason why he was still holding on. With my head buried in my dad's chest, crying uncontrollably, the hospice nurse rubbed my back and coached me on what to say and do to let my dad go so he could take his final breath. With everything in me with so much hurt and pain, I told my dad it was okay for him to go; the boys and I will be okay. I remember I kept telling him, "I promise daddy, I will be okay. I promise". It was not even a full minute later that he took his last breath and stopped breathing. At that very moment, I felt like someone took a knife and literally cut my heart out of my body. I cried. I screamed. I yelled. But none of that brought my dad, my best friend, back.

I just stayed at his side until I could not stay anymore and the funeral home came to take him away. I remember running behind the cart and the car until they shut that door and drove off with my dad's body. I was so hurt, devastated, and traumatized that I passed out. From that point forward, I did not want to be around anyone. Talk to anyone. I kept to myself a lot and stayed away from the house as much as I could. I was mad. I was angry. I could not believe that not only was my dad gone, but I was like, we just went through this, three times with my dad's brothers.

My mom, brothers, and I gave my dad the best homegoing and celebration of life that we could possibly give him. That was my first time experiencing the planning and preparing of a funeral. It was very hard, but we got through it by the strength and grace of God. I remember all the details of that day just like it happened yesterday. As we were getting ready to depart for the services, and my brothers and I were on the program to speak on behalf of our dad, I was lost for words. As much as I love my dad and as close as we were, I could not find the words to say because I was so heartbroken. My auntie, who is like my best friend and second mom, came into my room and comforted me and encouraged me and told me to just find a song in my heart to give me the peace and strength I needed to get through this. Taking my favorite auntie's advice, I found that song in my heart that not only brought me peace, it brought me strength, and joy in the days, weeks, and months that came afterward. But it was my reflection of my dad and what I sang at his celebration that best summed up my heart, feelings, and emotions.

"When peace like a river attendeth my way
When sorrows like sea billows roll
Whatever my lot, Thou hast taught me to say
It is well, it is well with my soul
It is well (it is well)

With my soul (with my soul)
It is well, it is well with my soul!"
That song was my testimony of the pain, grief, and sorrow I had experienced with my dad and the loss of three uncles within an eleven-month time frame. My dad's wisdom of getting back into the church, and connecting myself with a church body and a church family helped me to this point of even having the courage and faith to say "It is well with my soul!"

But what was the worst day of my life also became the best day of my life. The day we buried my dad was the exact same day I met my current husband. Even during sickness, death, and grieving, God was still watching over us. As believers and Christians, nothing is a "coincidence". My husband was not working his regular full-time job that day due to a severe bee sting. He was called by his part-time job to see, by chance, if he was already off to help with the funeral service of my dad. Due to his bee sting, he was not at his full-time job and was able to work his part-time job. He actually drove one of the family cars that my mom and brothers rode in. Matter of fact, I sat in the front seat next to him. On the way there, I had not noticed him. I didn't say anything as I was trying to prepare my heart, mind, and emotions for one of the worst days of my life. I remember as we were coming around the curve to the church, cars were everywhere. So many cars that you could see them from miles away from the church. The church parking lot and field were packed to capacity and extended to the next-door businesses. It brought tears of joy to our hearts to see how many people came out to remember my dad. There were so many people that many did not make it inside the church or the fellowship hall and had to leave. We felt such a burden lifted and a sense of relief from the numerous people and cars we saw there for my dad. You would have thought my dad was a Hollywood superstar. But we made it through the services and burial. After the burial, I did not want to be bothered or around anyone, so I went and sat in the car while I waited for my mom and brothers who were inside for the repass. I just felt so sad and alone and reality was kicking in that I was going back home and my dad would not be there, nor was he coming back. As I sat in the car, my sisters-in-law came and joined me. My oldest brother's wife was saying and doing all kinds of things to make me laugh including trying to bring my attention to the undertaker who was leaning on the car from the outside. I remember telling her that a man was the farthest thing from my mind and I know I prayed and asked God to not send anyone to me that was not from Him especially since I had just come out of a divorce from my second marriage.

My sister-in-law, being the humorous person she is, kept at it. She made jokes such as "Papa John sending you your next husband". Some of it

I cannot even repeat, as funny as it was. Of course, I ignored her at that moment, but appreciated her much later.

After we arrived back at the house and he said his normal speech to the families, he asked to talk to me outside. He shared with me the conversations he and my sister-in-law had outside. He also made me aware that he knew my dad and my dad had helped them out on funerals in the past. I believe that was the one and only thing that caught my attention and interest because he knew my dad. He came back over later that evening, and that was the first of many nights he came over. He was there for me, my mom, and my boys.

Our first date and hang-out spot was the Taverns on Main Street. In the beginning, we talked more about my dad and how he knew him more than anything else. The more we talked, the more I kept saying to myself, "This must be God and my daddy looking out for us". What was even more ironic, is that the more I got to know my current husband, the more he reminded me of my dad. He had a lot of my dad's ways and personality. It was almost too good to be true. I had to keep pinching myself to make sure I was not trapped in a dream. Those days turned into weeks, and those weeks turned into months. It gave my brothers and Godfather so much peace and joy knowing that even though dad was gone, there was a man around to look after me, my mom, and the boys. You would think after two marriages, I would be used to dating, but it was much different. The difference was I was still living at home and even though I was an adult, I had to respect my mom's house. Not only was I grown, but I was also finally finishing my studies to become a licensed clergy. Therefore, I could not date like everyone else. I had to carry myself in a manner that was pleasing to God and respectable to myself, my mom, and my boys. All of these things literally forced us to date, or as old folks would say and do, "court". It felt great having someone come and pick me up and take me out on dates. I felt like a young girl in high school because I literally had not "courted" anyone in this manner (the correct way) since I was in high school. This experience was totally different and unlike any others.

I was floating on "cloud nine" and enjoying all of my time with him that I forgot to do my annual physical and my first mammogram since turning forty. My birthday is always my reminder to do my annual physical and mammogram. Again, I was so happy and enjoying life after all of the pain and grief I experienced that I forgot to schedule my annual appointments. But by the end of March, my doctor's office reached out to me since they had not heard from me, which was unusual. So I scheduled my appointments for April 2015. I went in one spring morning for my routine mammogram. Less than 24-hours later they called me back and said they needed to do an ultrasound because of my dense breasts. A couple of days later I went in for the ultrasound, and once again I received a call less than 24-hours later requesting a biopsy. I am still floating on cloud nine from this man that came into my life and enjoying dating and being "courted", so I was not even worried or thinking about all the different tests I was doing. But then the unthinkable happened.

April 30, 2015, as I was driving into work from Sumter to Columbia. Talking to my new boo on my way to work, like I normally do. While we were talking, I noticed an incoming call from my doctor's office and asked him to hold on so I could click over to see what they needed. Here I am thinking they were calling me to tell me everything was negative, instead the nurse was asking for me to come into the doctor's office as soon as possible because my test results came back positive for breast cancer. Just when I thought Cancer had broken my heart four times already into a million pieces, here I was again facing this demon! Words can never begin to describe the emotions, the fear, the panic, and the heartbreak I experienced in that very moment of that phone call. Before I could call my mom, I called Jay back and told him what they said. I am sure by the time we got off that call, I had drained him as much as the call drained me. He stayed on the phone with me and talked with me until I made it to work. I told him I needed to get myself together before I could call my mom.

I went into work that morning feeling like all the air was just sucked from my body. It was taking everything in me to not show any emotions or let anyone know about the phone call I had just received. As I was walking to my desk after clocking in, my boss at the time was waiting for me to arrive at work and asked me into his office. So caught up in the phone call I had just received that I was not even caring or concerned about what he had to say. I went into his office and sat down and he went on to tell me how much he appreciates me and the good work that I have done over the years. I was hearing him but not hearing him because I was still caught up in my emotions from the phone call from my doctor's office. But he said something that not only caught my attention but helped me to snap out of the daze I was in. He told me that he was leaving the firm and he asked the firm to find another position for me so I could continue to work there. He probably thought I was crazy because I immediately started laughing out loud and thinking to myself "I am being punked!". So concerned about my appointment that afternoon I had to put aside everything else he was saying and bringing to my attention. I ended that conversation by letting him know I had a doctor's appointment that afternoon.

Thereafter, I went to my desk, called my mom and told her about the phone call, and asked her to come to Columbia and go with me. My mom's very close friend that we have known all my life, drove her to Columbia and we met at my job. They followed me to the doctor's office. I was so nervous. You would have thought I was waiting to see if I was pregnant or not. They finally called us to the back, and my doctor started from the beginning of the first test to the biopsy and explained everything to us.

The one thing that I remember, above all, is that he said he noticed I was almost 4 months late with my physical and that was probably a good thing because the breast cancer was on the onset and was just forming and it was barely a Stage 1. He went on further to say, had I completed my mammogram in January like I normally do, it would have been probably another year till the next mammogram that I would have discovered it. And by that time, the result and stage could have been different. At that moment, that very moment, I knew God had His hand on me and that everything was going to be okay. I reminded myself of that song in my heart, "It is Well with my Soul! Needless to say, I was so concerned about the diagnosis I totally forgot about the changes that were getting ready to take place with my employer after my boss left the firm. The next day there was a letter on my desk from my employer advising me that they were not going to find another position for me and my employment would be ending in two weeks, my boss's last day. There are not enough words in the dictionary to find nor describe that moment. I was speechless. I was hurt. I was scared! I remember clocking out and going into the parking lot and just screaming and crying. So much pain and sadness begin to be released from my inner gut. I could not believe this was happening to me. I needed my health insurance to be able to do my surgery and radiation. I was a single parent with limited income due to all the deductions I had coming out of my check for health insurance and other benefits. I just kept asking myself "what am I going to do?".

As I was getting myself together, our office manager was returning from lunch and saw me in the parking lot upset and she began to pray with me, pray for me, sing to me, and reminded me of God's word. We sat in the parking lot and we talked for a long time as she reminded me who I was in Christ Jesus. It was that very moment I remembered the song in my heart, "It is well with my soul!" and began to sing it over and over and over again until I was at peace. I just went on as planned with all of my appointments to prepare for my surgery and continued to come to work every day trusting God because it was all well with my soul. The day before it was scheduled to be my last day at the firm, the managing partner from the firm met with me and informed me that they found a position for me and that if I was interested, I could continue to work and maintain my employment and benefits there. When I say nobody but God, it was truly nobody but God. Once again, God reminded me that He got me!

Even after God turned that entire work situation around in my favor, the more I tried to stay positive and think positive, the more the devil played with my thoughts and my mind. The more I reminded myself of the God I served and believed in, the more the devil reminded me of what I just went through with cancer concerning my dad and three uncles. Also during this diagnosis and genetic testing, I discovered that my grandfather, my dad's father, was the first black male in South Carolina to be diagnosed with breast cancer in the mid '70s and possibly contributed to his death when I was a toddler. After finding that information, I made a declaration and confession over my life that I was going to break the generational curse of cancer. Not only over my life, but over my children and my children's children. I went boldly before God reminding Him of His word and confessing that cancer will not hurt anyone else in my family and I pleaded the blood of Jesus not only over my body and health, but for every family member. I spoke life that we will not lose anyone else in our family to cancer IN JESUS NAME!

At this point, I had to put all of my emotions aside and realize this was spiritual warfare and I had to fight back with the word of God. It was challenging because the more I confessed and believed, the more the devil planted thoughts and images of death in my mind. But I refused to give in to his scheme and thoughts. My mom, my children, and Jay were there with me every step of the way. Even before a proposal and a marriage, Jay proved not only his love for me, but that he could love me in sickness and in health. We had not been together a year and we were dealing with this after all the tragedy and heartbreak my family was still healing and recovering from.

Now, this is strike five of Cancer breaking our hearts and this became very personal for me. It took every strength and all the faith inside of me to get through this journey while still grieving the loss and absence of my best friend, my dad. But I handled it like that champion God created me to be and my dad raised me in the confidence to have.

After a lumpectomy in May 2015, removing 40% of my right breast, followed by eight weeks of radiation every morning from 8 am- 8 30am before having to work eight hours straight, followed by a pill I would have to take for the next five years. I conquered and survived Stage I DCIS breast cancer. Nobody but God! By September 2015, I was cancer free and my breast cancer journey was over! At least, that is what I thought was the final outcome.

As life for me continued after cancer broke my heart once again, I noticed my body was not the same. As I tried to move on with life, as it was before the breast cancer diagnosis, my body would not let me be great. Something just was not right but I could not figure it out. The next month was my husband's birthday month. I wanted to do something very special for him for his birthday for being an awesome support system for me during my breast cancer journey. Most men would have checked out and considered this to be too much, especially for someone they were just dating. But God did not send me 'that type of man'. But instead, one who was caring, loving, and very supportive. I tell him all the time now, that he actually was showing to me and proving to me, even before we were engaged and married, that he would love me in sickness and in health.

What was so ironic about our relationship at that time is that even though we were single, all the couples we were close to and spent a lot of our time with were all married. In fact, we were the only two singles out of the group (haha). We had some great role models, of different ages and backgrounds while we were dating. I planned for a few of us to go back to my old stomping grounds in Greenville, South Carolina. Greenville was my home for eleven years and it has by far been the best place I have ever lived. I missed living there. I planned a perfect weekend with the man I love and the people who were closest to our hearts.

Little did I know a celebration and a well-planned weekend to celebrate and show my appreciation for my husband turned out to be an engagement weekend. Yes, we officially got engaged that weekend and I was very excited to marry my best friend, who was there for me through two heartbreaks in my life caused by cancer–losing my dad, and then being diagnosed with breast cancer.

To me, this was a true love story that I never thought could happen to me again. I felt as if my guardian angel, my dad, was still taking care of me and looking out for me. My husband and my dad had a lot of ways and similarities that it was almost scary! (LOL) But God ordained and sent my husband just for me and I thank God daily for blessing me with someone who loved me through so much hurt and pain caused by Cancer.

Now that I was officially engaged and ready to marry my best friend, we began to start planning our wedding. Since this was not our first marriage, we planned a very simple but elegant and beautiful beach wedding with our immediate family and closest friends. I love the beach. It is one of my favorite places I love to go just to relax, relate and release all of the cares and troubles of this world.

April 23, 2016, I became Mrs. Ross and we began our new life together with our new blended family, four boys, and two girls. I felt so blessed that God loved me so much that He gave me a husband and bonus children as a blessing to me despite all of the hurt and pain I went through caused by cancer. As life for me began as Mrs. Ross, it was an adjustment to being a wife again, learning about my bonus children, and prioritizing everything with work, commuting, and being a wife and mother. Keep in mind that my body was still continuing to go through a lot of changes and adjustments after the breast cancer journey. Even though I was cancer-free, I was required to take a pill every night and it seemed like the longer I was taking that pill, the more my body felt like it was changing. I literally felt like my body was aging and fast-forwarding about twenty to thirty years. I remember complaining to my oncologist and kept telling them that something was not right.

As days turned into weeks and weeks turned into months, still, no one could tell me what was going on other than telling me "it's just the side effects from your medicine". These days, weeks, and months had now taken us into the fall–October. It was the first Sunday in October of 2016 and I woke up that morning not feeling well. I felt like I was hit by a truck and the entire right side of my body felt numb and very different. I remember not doing much that day and went to bed that night with a very bad headache and sharp pain in my right arm and shoulder. Sometime during the night, before it was time to prepare for work and school, I remember having an out-of-body experience I could not even explain and felt as if I had no control over my body. I remember trying to get up and could not. I remember trying to scream out for Caleb and could not. I tried calling my mom, as Jay had already left for work, and the thoughts in my head would not come out as words to talk to my mom to let her know something was not right and something was going on. My mom immediately knew something was not right and she not only came right over but called 9-1-1.

After that, all I remember is the doctor telling my mom and husband that I had what was called a TIA stroke. Not able to talk without a slur, walking with a limp, and holding my right arm as if it felt like a hundred pounds, I spent a week in the hospital with doctors puzzled and trying to figure out what contributed to me having a TIA stroke. I was even transferred from one hospital to another hospital that was more experienced in neurology to help give me the answers I needed as to why. On the last day of being released, the head neurologist at the second hospital, where I was now being treated, gave me some information and knowledge that caught me by surprise. In "his opinion", he felt the stroke was caused by a little stress and anxiety, but his biggest concern was that I was very overweight for the pill I was taking every night as a cancer blocker. He advised me of all the side effects of the medicine. And "stroke" was one of the primary side effects–especially with being overweight for that type of medicine.

Of course, I was in shock and this was all new information to me. The first thing I was thinking was why my oncologist did not inform me of this? Of course, I was instructed to follow up with my oncologist after being released. A few days after being released, my mom and I did my follow-up with my oncologist. At this point, I was not happy and felt like my doctor did not educate me, nor did they have my best interest at heart. I kept complaining to my doctor that something was not right, but I was always told nothing was wrong, it was just the side effects. I went on to inform them of what I was told before I was discharged and the response was "Did you not read the information pamphlet that came with your medicine?" At this point, I'm like are you kidding me?! It was a good thing my speech was still impaired and prevented me from saying things due to my physical impairment. I felt as if my oncologist was blaming me for what happened. In my opinion, I felt like it was my oncologist's responsibility to "inform me" of the side effects of the medicine that was prescribed for me. Yes, it may have been my responsibility to read the pamphlet but it was also my doctor's responsibility to inform me of all of the pros and cons of anything being prescribed to me.

I remember leaving there feeling helpless and defeated. I was taken off the medicine and was informed to find a primary care doctor and focus on getting better with my speech and physical impairments on my right side. I made getting better and healthier my priority. At that moment, I realized that I had to advocate for myself and my health. I also learned that you cannot depend on and rely on doctors. So even though I left my follow-up appointment feeling defeated, I also left feeling encouraged and motivated to take better care of myself. As a family, we got through that moment and experience. It was an eye-opener to a lot of things, and made me put a lot of things regarding life into perspective. I learned to appreciate life more by making myself my number one priority. Of course, as with many of us, we always start off hard and well but with the many roles we play in life and the many hats we wear, we always seem to get off course with making self a priority.

As life continued, I moved on as a wife, mother, sister, auntie, cousin, friend, and employee. I was trying to learn how to balance not just my life, but my priorities. There were times when something required more of my attention and time than others. I tried my best to manage and prioritize it all so nothing would go lacking. One thing I learned is that as a woman, we don't get breaks. We have to demand them and just take them. As women, there is something that has to always be done and most of the time we lose ourselves and take better care of others than we do ourselves. As I began 2018 with a new attitude and mindset, once again my body was not allowing me to be great. But this time, I did not have a pill to blame it on. I found myself feeling tired all the time. I noticed that my legs and feet hurt a lot and felt very heavy. As time kept passing by, I noticed I developed this dry cough I could not shake and the cough would be worse at night. Something was not right. Staying busy, there was always something I had to do with work, home, kids, and husband, that I did not take the time to go and see a doctor. Once again, the days turned into weeks and months and time was passing by. I was taking care of everyone and everything else but Tamekia. The more time passed by, the more my body kept giving me warning signs. And the more I kept ignoring them because I did not "make the time". There were so many demands and expectations from me that I was afraid and hesitant to take the time I needed for me to figure out what was going on because I knew that any time I took for myself, something or someone would be lacking. I have spent my entire life putting everything and everyone before myself.

It was eight months later, August of 2018, and I was driving home from work. As I was crossing the bridge between Columbia and Sumter, I noticed that my right hand began to swell and my right arm was tightening. Of course, the first thing I thought was, "not a stroke again". By the time I got home, I could not even take my arm out of my clothing. I started taking Benadryl and Tylenol and I remember my mom and husband questioned me as to what I ate that day, and what I might have done that may have contributed to what was going on. We even came up with the assumption that maybe something bit me. The swelling eventually went down but a couple of hours later it came back. This time it was very painful. At this point, I went to the ER. They ran some tests, did an ultrasound and other tests, and could not determine what was causing the swelling. I was discharged with "lymphoedema" and was told to follow up with my oncologist. But that could not be right because I did not have any lymph nodes removed during my lumpectomy, so how could the ER misdiagnose me like that.

The next morning I called my oncologist office and told them what was going on and they saw me right away. Unfortunately, I was not greeted with concern by my oncologist. Instead they fussed at me. I was ridiculed like a child for still not having a primary doctor and reminding me that they were not my primary doctor and what I should have done instead of calling them. At this point, I was more concerned about what was going on with my body rather than a debate with my oncologist. After going through all of the preliminaries, I was taken into a room for an ultrasound. Thereafter, I was immediately rushed to the ER where I was admitted into the hospital and treated for a blood clot in my right jugular vein. I can't begin to describe the fear I was experiencing at that moment and during that time. I thought this part of my life was over and I should not be going through any of this, especially since I was cancer-free. I kept asking God, "why was this happening to me?" I spent three nights and four days in the hospital and was sent home. I was prescribed blood thinners.

Once again, I went on with life completing all of my priorities and expectations while trying to understand and still find answers to unanswered questions. One month after being on the blood thinners, I was starting not to feel like myself again and my body was going through changes again. This time I was having shortness of breath on top of all of the other issues I started having at the beginning of the year with bone pain. I called my oncologist and kept calling and complaining and finally was able to get an appointment. Once again, I was fussed at and ridiculed about calling my oncologist office versus finding a primary doctor. I explained that it was hard being able to get a primary because no one was taking new patients. Due to the shortness of breath and because of the blood clot, I was immediately scheduled for a CT scan of my chest. As I waited in the room for the results, I just started praying and seeking God like I never have in my life. My oncologist walked in and told me that there was a spot on my lungs and they needed to do a full-body PETScan right away.

Remaining calm and unfamiliar with all of these medical terms, I just did as I was told. A couple of days later, I completed my PETScan. Two days later we received a call that there was a "red" area that lit up on my tailbone that required a biopsy. So once again, immediately after the PETScan, a biopsy of my right tail bone was completed. Thereafter, my husband and I were scheduled for a follow-up with my oncologist. Just a couple of days later, my husband met me at my oncologist office. I remember we sat in the lobby and in the office just laughing and talking; not worried at all about the results because we were confident that everything was okay. My oncologist eventually walked in, spoke, and said with no remorse or using any kind of bedside manners, "Your biopsy report came back as Stage IV breast cancer". As my oncologist continued to go on and talk despite the fact that I literally lost it. I fell off the table and went into a hysterical panic attack. I heard nothing else after "Stage IV ". I remember my husband kept telling the doctor to stop, and wait a minute as he was trying to help me get myself together. I finally got myself together as the oncologist continued to talk, and all I heard and all I remember to this day "Stage IV" and "there is no cure for it and we will do our best to try to treat you as long as we can." November 5, 2018 cancer broke my heart again. I remember telling my husband, my pastor, and everyone that I talked to "I will not accept this!" Not only was I not going to accept it, but I wanted a second opinion. I felt as if my oncologist never fought for me, nor had they advocated for me. They just "treated" me. And that was unacceptable. I could not put my life in the hands of someone who saw me and treated me as an assigned account number rather than a human being. I wanted and needed someone who was going to fight for my life with me.

Thanks to Facebook, I remember one of my college alumni shared numerous posts regarding her breast cancer journey and how she had to go somewhere else for her treatments. I reached out to her on Facebook and she immediately called me and gave me some information regarding the Cancer

Treatment Centers of America. I shared with her some of my experiences with my oncologist and we discovered that even though we had a different oncologist, we both were going to the same cancer center. Talking to her just confirmed I needed to go somewhere else.

In addition to reaching out to my college alumni, I also reached out to my classmate who was also a cousin, as I was informed that she took her husband there as well who was also a classmate and cousin to me. I reached out to her and she gave me a lot of information as well and spoke very highly of the cancer treatment centers.

While I was looking into going there, my oncologist put me on a pill to take. So many days on and so many days off. There was no discussion about chemo, radiation, or anything else. I had questions about what to do, what not to do, what to eat, and what not to eat, and was never given a direct answer nor the information or knowledge that I needed for this diagnosis. I remember becoming very depressed and sad. My mind and thoughts took me back to 2013-2014 of what our family went through regarding my dad and his brothers. My mind, my heart, and my thoughts became so overwhelming I did not know how to comprehend everything that was going on.

That following Monday I finally made the decision and reached out to Cancer Treatment Centers. I completed the online application and less than thirty minutes from hitting the "submit button" a representative contacted me. I was impressed by them from the start. Even during the process and while speaking to a representative, I began to feel relieved. By that Wednesday, my insurance had approved everything and we were scheduled.

As we were waiting for the upcoming appointment, I remember being home alone one evening. I started to listen to gospel on pandora. The more the gospel music played, the more each song began to minister to my heart, my soul, and my spirit. Probably by the fifth song, I was laying on the floor in a cradle position, just crying and hollering to the top of my lungs. I cried as I have never cried in my entire life. I would cry. I would pray. I would sing. I would cry. I would pray. I would sing. Then I began to just call the name "Jesus!". The more I called His name, the more I felt a "lifting". The more I called His name, the more the heaviness became lighter. The more I called His name, the more encouraged I became. After spending hours in His presence, I got up off the floor with a new attitude and a new mindset and the word that I got off that floor with, has kept me till this day. That word is…Faith!

From that day forward, I started filling my spirit with sermons, prayers, scriptures, and everything that reminded me of who God is and what He promised me. Even as a licensed minister of the gospel, I can honestly admit that my faith was shaken. Not only was my faith shaken, but the past four years of being licensed, this moment and journey also reminded me that a title does not exempt us from life experiences. We can get so hung up on the titles and existence that we forget to live. Not just live, but in Him, we live and have our being.

I not only forgot to make Tamekia a priority and take care of Tamekia, but I also was so busy and consumed with everything and everyone else that I did not make my relationship with Him a priority. We sometimes get so focused on making sure we go to church, bible study, and do everything asked of us that we disconnect ourselves from the main source of where all of our help comes from. It is not that I did not want to spend time with Him, but I did not make Him my priority because, by the time I was finished taking care of everything and everyone else, I did not make room for Him because I was too tired or fell asleep every time I tried.

But this time, yes this time, I made Jesus my first priority because I knew Jesus and my faith in Him was the only thing I can depend on and rely on to get me through this journey of my life.

In December of 2018 my husband and I made our initial trip to Cancer Treatment Centers of America in Newnan, Georgia. I can honestly say the three days we were there, I learned more in three days about breast cancer in general and my current diagnosis more than what I knew in the three years of being diagnosed for the first time in April of 2015. They explained and broke everything down to the point that I understood it all and had no unanswered questions. We learned more about my diagnosis from that visit than from the other visits I had back in South Carolina. We understood the biopsy results, what type of breast cancer I had, where it had metastasized, and how they could treat it. My doctor asked me one question, "Mrs. Ross, do you want to live?" Of course, I replied, yes, absolutely. He then explained to me why there was no cure for Stage IV but also reminded me and encouraged me of the numerous women with the same diagnosis that had beat the odds and were still fighting and living life and that the end result was up to me and God. It would be based on the work I was willing to put in to fight and live.

I was informed it was a major lifestyle adjustment, but there was medicine to help me with the adjustments and I had to do my part along with the medicine doing its part. I informed them that I was willing to do the work and that I was ready to fight. We left that Wednesday to return home and informed our family of everything. I felt such a peace that I have not had since my dad passed away. Knowledge is powerful and getting an understanding can change your life and your attitude.

Even though it was a lot of information to take in and digest, CTCA educated me on my HER2+ diagnosis that spread outside of my right breast to my bones with spots (possible metastases) on my liver, lymph nodes, and chest that they would monitor regularly through quarterly CT scans and PETScans every six months. I also discovered that it was hormone and estrogen-driven and how certain things over the course of my life contributed to and increased my chances such as being on birth control most of my life. We don't realize how chemicals, toxins and our environmental exposure contributes to breast cancer.

We were only home four days before we were on the road again back to Newnan, Georgia. The first day we had the surgery for my port to be put in and the next day I started nine and a half hours of three different types of the harshest chemos. On day three I did my fluids that morning and got my patch and we were on the road headed home with all of the instructions and my meds until the next visit in three weeks. Wednesday night we arrived home and Thursday morning both my husband and I were back at work.

My first day at work was fine. I was nervous and tired as I did not know what to expect. But I made it through the day and drove home after work and went straight to bed. Friday came and we did the same thing. But by the time I got home from work that Friday my body was beginning to experience things unknown. I became nauseous, very weak, and lost my appetite. By Monday I had an uncontrollable and burning diarrhea that lasted three days. By the following weekend, I felt like myself again minus the low energy and no appetite.

We continued this routine of leaving on Sundays, chemo on Mondays and Tuesdays, driving back home Tuesday nights, and back to work on Wednesdays. This went on until May 2019. There were days when my legs would shake. Times where I felt like my body was being electrocuted. I lost my hair and was bald for a year. My skin became very dark. I hid my black nails behind my pink fingernail polish. Some of my toenails began to pop off. I started out at 210 pounds and was down to 155. There were so many changes in my life and in my body. It may have broken my heart but it did not break my faith. By June 2019, I was down to one chemo treatment every three weeks. I went from 9 ½ hours to 3 hours of chemo. Every six months I have my CT scans, bone density, and PETScan. Every three months I have to do an echocardiogram to ensure the ongoing treatment is not affecting my heart. I can't even begin to describe my nerves every time I have to repeat these tests. But I allowed my Faith to overshadow any fears that tried to take over my mind and thoughts. Psalms 91 and Dr. Cindy Trimm's "Healing Prayer" has gotten me through a lot of moments to calm my fears and activate my faith. My husband and my youngest son, Caleb, have seen parts of my journey that no one has any clue about. The times I yelled and screamed in the middle of the night from the charlie horses in my calves that felt like someone was taking a knife and cutting through my bones. But I remained faith strong. The times when I lost my bowels or urinated on myself uncontrollably; I remained faith strong. The numerous nights I was afraid to be in the house by myself or sleep in the room alone; I remained faith strong. The times my bones were in so much pain and so stiff that they had to help me out of the bed, to the bathroom, and even wipe me. But I remained Faith Strong.

"And we know that in all things God works for the good of those who love him, who have been called according to his purpose." Romans 8:28 Even though Cancer has broken my heart numerous times since 2012, it strengthened my faith and helped me to find my purpose. Even through cancer, it is working out for my good. As a two-time breast cancer survivor, I never knew or heard about metastatic breast cancer until I was diagnosed a second time November 5, 2018. During this second diagnosis, I have learned so much more regarding breast cancer, especially among African American Women.

I, along with my co-founder, Tammey Davis, found this to be true when we were both diagnosed with metastatic breast cancer in our mid 40's in 2018. We both were very shocked and concerned as to how and why this could happen to us at a very early age. The difference between Tammey and I was the fact that it was my second diagnosis of breast cancer whereas it was her first diagnosis. Imagine being diagnosed the very first time and being told it was Stage IV and there is no cure for the disease.

Stage IV Metastatic Breast Cancer brought Tammey and me together, but our faith in God made us sisters and helped us find our purpose in life through the pain and hurt of this diagnosis. I remember sharing with Tammey one night over dinner that God has a purpose and a plan for the diagnosis and what we are going through. I shared with Tammey how God kept telling me "this is not about you, but for someone else and He will get the Glory". To my surprise, God was telling Tammey the same thing. From that moment on, I began to pray and seek God like never before as to my purpose and His plan for my life through this second diagnosis, now Stage IV. By the next time we met for dinner and our circle grew with other pink sisters who began meeting with us Fridays for dinner, I shared with them the vision God gave me to start a support group as well as write a book. They all were very encouraging and gave me the motivation I needed to "write the vision and make it plain.". They not only encouraged me, but offered assistance to make it happen.

So, what started out as a few women coming together every Friday night for dinner to fellowship, encourage and support each other turned into a support group for women, faith strong. I immediately became very transparent and open about my journey and began sharing with everyone on Facebook. The more I shared, the more women reached out to me and the more people from the community made others aware of me. I in return connected them to Faith Strong, Inc. and the other BREASTies. Our support group has reached a multitude of women as far as California. So here I am. I am here and it is by the grace of God. I am walking by Faith and not by a diagnosis. Every day I wake up, I give God back His word of what He promised me, "Tamekia, your Faith has healed you!" (Mark 5:34) "Tamekia, this sickness is not unto death, but for the Glory of God" (John 11:4) Even after three of our BREASTies did not receive their healing on this side of heaven, yes it has broken my heart to pieces but it did not break my faith.

There are some things I have experienced since November 5, 2018 that broke my heart and broke me to my knees, but they did not break my faith. I had to overcome night terrors, and night fears, and go through therapy, but it did not break my faith. There were times when I did not have the money to make the trip to Atlanta every three weeks but it did not break my faith and God always provided. My medical expenses and travel expenses exceed my monthly income but it never broke my faith. There were mornings and times I could barely walk and the pain was so unbearable but it never broke my faith. The winter and cold months are the hardest on my body and I hurt the most, but it never broke my faith. I have family and there are people I once called "friends" that I knew would be there for me to support me. There are some I still have yet to hear from them to this day or receive any type of support but, it never broke my faith. Sickness and disease does not exempt how people will treat you, talk about you, hurt you or disappoint you. I went from being able to wear five-inch stilettos most of my life to only being able to wear special shoes, which broke my heart, but not my faith. People know I am living with a Stage IV metastatic breast cancer to the bones and have a lot of challenges and physical limitations and don't care and will treat you and talk to you without any consideration, but, it never broke my faith. I have been talked about, disrespected, mistreated, bullied, lied to, lied on, misunderstood, fighting more with the world than fighting for my life, but it never broke my faith. I have learned that the weapons may be formed but they will not prosper.

Don't just tell people you love them, show them you love them. There is ALWAYS a need for someone affected by breast cancer, especially if they are stage IV and it is ongoing. Don't ask, just do it! Too many people have given up because they did not have the support they needed to keep fighting. The card you send, the phone call you make, the unexpected visit you may pay, and the monetary support you give, may just be the very thing that someone needs to save their life and encourage them to keep fighting and not give up. When we take care of God's people, God will take care of us! November 5, 2018 will mark four years of my stage IV metastatic breast cancer journey, and I am still faith strong and standing on the promises of God. Thanks be to God who gives me the victory through Christ Jesus that I don't look like what I been through. To date, I have completed over fifty treatments and I continue to travel to Cancer Treatment Centers of America in Newnan, Georgia for treatment, scans, and repeating the cycle. I wake up every morning taking eight bills and before going to bed, take an additional ten more pills. And sometimes even more if I am having any complications. But guess what? I won't complain because my good days are still outweighing my bad days because God has been just that good to me. My God is bigger than cancer and my faith outweighs my fears.

As this journey continues, I continue to build the vision that God gave me to help the people of God who are affected by breast cancer. It is not about me or what I am going through, but it's all about Him, and what He can do if we simply just have faith. I am just living my life out loud and on purpose to be a representation of Him on this earth (as it is in heaven). If I can help somebody, then my living, my diagnosis will not be in vain. Cancer broke my heart, but it did not break my Faith because I am FULLY persuaded by what God has promised, He is also able to perform. (Romans 4:21)

My favorite poet Dr. Maya Angelou stated, *"People will forget what you said, people will forget what you did, but people will never forget how you make them feel"*

I would like to thank each of the following individuals for praying for me, constantly sowing into me financially to assist me in traveling to Atlanta every three weeks for treatment, and with my ongoing medical expenses. I thank you and pray God richly blesses you for ALL that you have done for me with my ongoing medical expenses.

Anthriest & Frances D. Hill	Dr. Kimberly Green
Keith & Angelia "Angie" Neal	Dr. Bernice Heyward Mullins
Auntie Paulette Morgan	Pastor Linda Speed
Auntie Tryphenia Speed	Martha Grant Scott
Nikkita "Nikki" Lewis	Burnette Shutt & McDaniel Law Firm
Karren Hill Gordon	Al & Cheryl Squire
Antonio & Jennifer Ray	Cousins Alvin & Janet King
Stephanie Grant Brown	Attorney Nekki Shutt
Tonya Wilson Moten	Jason T. Mahoney
Johnny & Gaylinda Phillips	St. Luke A.M.E. Church
Helen Pinckney Nixon	Victory Church
Cory Wilson	Tywanda Pringle Hurt

Pastor Terrence and First Lady Shaunya Murrill

The Independent Unbroken ......H
Tammey Davis

Someone once asked me, "Who is Tammey". Well, I laughed at that question. Not because it was funny, but because I was not sure if the person was ready to receive who I was. For you see, I am the definition of a "Strong Black Woman". I always held down multiple jobs, raised my kids, endured a divorce, was always full of energy, and never allowed any dirt to stay under my feet. I was just that girl you could rock with, hanging out on a weekend and the one that would be with you in prayer and at your call when you needed me. I just love life, and people, and enjoy a good time. And I was always willing to put in the work for what I needed and wanted. You can sum it up by saying, I am independent and unbroken. And I am not about games.

I have never been afraid of anything, but life has a way of "testing" your commitment to God and your realness. Well, in 2018, my test came. In 2018 something about me started changing. I did a self- mammogram and at that moment, I realized something was wrong because my breast started getting heavy. I went to the doctor, but they could not find anything wrong. I kept going back and forth but continued to receive the same thing. Each time, something different would impact my body. My hair started coming out, my breast continued to get heavy, and they could not find anything wrong. My body continued to endure even more changes. I started losing weight, my body shape changed, and I became a 42 DD–my girls got real HEAVY. When my hair started coming out in patches, I knew something was wrong. However, I went back to the doctor again, and even my lab work came back clear. In September 2018, I did another self-exam and found a lump. Upon finding a lump I made an appointment to see the gynecologist. He noticed the lump also that Wednesday and scheduled for me to do a mammogram. Once I had the mammogram and biopsy, I received a call that changed my life forever. My test results came back positive. After going through a long hard divorce at the age of 38 with two sons, I got diagnosed with HER2+ stage 3a breast cancer.

After getting a diagnosis, they told me that it was rapidly spreading and it was already in my lymph nodes. We had to move fast on the treatment. By October 1st I was getting a port put in for treatment. I started my first chemo session on October 12th at 9 o'clock in the morning. 72 hours after my first treatment, my body started changing. I lost my hair and I ended up in the hospital. My body did not accept the first chemo treatment. I had to complete treatment every two weeks, and it was always on a Thursday. My first treatment lasted eight hours and my second treatment lasted seven hours.

After the second treatment, I felt really ill, to the point that the doctor didn't understand what was going on. So they gave me the third treatment. That third treatment landed me in the hospital with bruises from the inside. My body was burning from the inside out. I was having difficulty with my legs. Different teams of doctors were called to come and see if they recognized what was going on with my body. They came, and no one could tell me what was going on. It was on that day that I decided to meet with three young ladies that have been diagnosed with cancer and were going through similar changes in their life. After meeting with them, I decided to call cancer treatment centers. I got there. They ran the test again to make sure that I was receiving the right type of treatment for my cancer and also they noticed that I was having an allergic reaction to it. I was rejecting the Herceptin that was given because they were pushing the treatment hard and my body decided to reject that type of treatment. So every time I received the treatment, it would land me in the hospital because my body couldn't dispose of it and I was having an inside allergic reaction when I got to Atlanta in January. They told me that I had to have a double mastectomy and that the tumor did shrink since it was first discovered. They went ahead and scheduled me to start going to Atlanta and to start going to CTCA every three weeks instead of every two weeks for treatment. It was at that point they said my markers were down. My numbers were low enough for me to have a double mastectomy. I had a double mastectomy back at home, not in CTCA. While doing a double mastectomy, which had actually been a success, I went into cardiac arrest. I had too much medicine in my system and my heart couldn't fight off what was going on. I stayed in ICU. I remained in an introverted coma for a week and a half. After a week and a half, I was able to get back to CTCA to see the doctor. Then the doctor down there told me I had to do treatment and radiation. I had to do a total of 45 rounds of radiation, along with chemo. I would have to complete radiation treatment Monday through Friday for 15 minutes at a time. The radiation burnt me so bad my whole torso became unrecognizable with blisters, just like those you get from a burn. I fought through it. I fought hard. I tried to stay strong through it all, like in the Bible, where they say you go through the flood and the rain and the fire. My body went through all three within six months At my second set of scans after surgery that's when they noticed a spot outside of where the original cancer started from. Once they found cancer somewhere else in your body that's when they diagnosed you with Stage 4 with a spot that is no longer there, but I still had to do the treatment after not having a support of a male in my life. I now have a boyfriend and we are reconnecting to the point that I had to deal with some issues with my body changing. The way I look. The way I feel. But once you reconnect with yourself, it makes a difference in your life and how you perceive dealing with or having been diagnosed with cancer. You get to reconnect with yourself! You get to know the woman who survived breast cancer. Take her out for a glass of wine and get to know her and how she thinks and feels. You might be thinking about how you have pain, or how you can't wear that one shirt you used to love because it doesn't fit right anymore. Or worried about how your breasts are gonna look, let alone feel, even in the eyes and arms of your true love. Get to know yourself and those deep thoughts and feelings. When you are in survival mode (aka When you are in survival mode aka Fight or Flight) you are in warrior mode and tired as all get out. Naturally, your guard is up, so pleasure is not even on your radar. Day to day in survival mode of just getting all the things done and managing your pain on top of it? That's a lot going on. In survival mode, it's easy to put all kinds of self-care to the side—for later. The same thing with intimacy, it's not really where I am yet. I'm sure we'll get there someday. Something to be aware of is your threshold. If you're having a very busy day, feel overwhelmed, and stuck in survival mode. Be in tune and aware of yourself; knowing this may not be a good day to try something new with your partner. I would schedule a DATE NIGHT! If you get to the place where you're comfortable being intimate with your partner again, but you experience vaginal pain, that can be addressed as well. I have gone through three scar release and pelvic floor therapy sessions to help. Consider talking to your OBGYN about ideas or suggestions. They would also be the ones who can give you a PT script for pelvic floor work. There is also the possibility that menopause could be affecting your pain with sex as well. All kinds of lubes and information exist that could make this enjoyable for you again. It's important to remember to work with your pain and not push through it. This can create bracing that brings on the fight or flight response and puts pleasure on the back burner.

Well, after my journey, the question was presented again, "Who is Tammey"? Well, the answer is still the same. However, I have evolved to more than I was before. Despite the diagnosis, I am an entrepreneur, engaged in my community, and serving my country. God said what I am going to take you through, is not for me, but for someone else. That's why I must keep fighting and you must as well.

See I view my diagnosis as a fighter in the boxing ring. As long as I practice what I have learned, condition myself, stay inside the ring, pay attention to my opponent, apply my techniques, and fight with perseverance, I am destined to win. Every day that we get up, there will be something that will try to attack our existence (our mind, body, and spirit). However, I need you to stay in the ring and stay fighting. Anything that comes your way— FIGHT! When you have nothing left—just FIGHT.

See, I am still in the ring. And I am in this ring for a reason. And when the championship badge of honor is given, my name shall reign.

This is my fight, but it is not who I Am…for I am Tammey Davis, "The Independent Unbroken ……H".

Another Hurtful Shocker
Dr. Bernice Mullins

On June 17, 2019, I lost the love of my life after 42 years of marriage. Another hurtful shocker transpired just four months later. On October 30, 2019, my grandson, Darrell "Ajay's", 18th birthday, I was told that I have cancer. My sister, Martha, and I sat quietly as the kind and gentle doctor, Dr. Henry Moses, told me that I have breast cancer that had spread to the lymph nodes. I could not breathe for a moment. As we walked out of the doctor's office, I felt the Lord holding me together. I heard his voice as I got into my truck and began to head home. I heard him say, "you have this, this is for my glory, and I am with you, do not fret or fear". I started to look around in the dark to see if someone else was in the truck with me. Martha drove her car and was not with me. I was the last patient that was seen by the doctor and it was dark when we left his office.

As I continued home, I found a peace that was not normal. I was four months into the grief of losing Roger and here it is, on my grandchild's birthday, I have cancer. I never shed a tear at first. I did not cry with the doctor and with my sister, Martha. She was so hurt, and I saw pain and compassion in her eyes. When I got home, I told my children. They were so upset and began to shed tears. I assured them that everything was going to be fine; I told them that God told me everything was going to be alright. We went on and celebrated Ajay's birthday with his favorite meal and cake. We agreed to not tell the grandchildren at that time. We all were still missing my husband, their father, and grandfather, Roger, so much. And I did not want to put a damper on Ajay's 18th birthday.

That night as with most other nights, I got on my knees and I prayed. The tears flowed profusely. I guess the prognosis of cancer and missing my husband was settling in on me and was more than I could bear. The grief dominated my mind and I wept to the Lord because I did not have my husband to comfort me, to hold me, to tell me that God will take care of me. God had told this to me earlier but the flesh longs for comfort. I remembered crying so much that I could not breathe. I had to take short breaths to settle down. The word of the Lord came to me again and began to minister to me. I felt God's presence calming me down.

From that night onward, I prayed, cried, prayed, cried, and wept, calling out for Jesus Christ my savior. One thing was for sure, I hurt over not having my soulmate more than cancer. I had peace about cancer. My doctor and others that had cancer assured me that so much had changed with chemotherapy and technology. The journey was not easy, but it could have been worse. I had my Lord, Jesus Christ, with me each step of the way. God gave me a spiritual daughter, Tameka Hunter Ross, who helped me in my walk with cancer. She has stage 4 cancer but lives a happy, kind, and resourceful life helping others. She founded a breast cancer support group to help anyone that needed love and support. Through this diagnosis, I have met some of the nicest and most humble women I ever dreamed of coming into contact with in this breast cancer support group and at the cancer treatment center. The world is fighting and conflicting with each other over politics and these ladies and men are fighting to live. At the cancer treatment center, everyone's plight is different, but the ultimate goal is to live and feel better. My ultimate goal is to live and represent Jesus Christ! And to testify of His healing powers and deliverance.

I have had so many people quote scriptures to me as a way to be done with this pain already. As stated, not only did I have to come through the recent death of my husband, but I was also diagnosed with breast cancer 4 months later. I had to endure harsh chemotherapy which took all of my hair, surgery, and radiation along with grief. I will admit that the grief's hurt was far worse than the diagnosis of cancer and its horrible journey. Regardless of what I was hearing, I had to believe the Word of God, and that Word must germinate in me before I could begin to walk in it. The one thing Roger would say is "going there shouldn't tell been there how to get there." Many people are in over their heads in understanding how the early phases of grief felt. I was in love with my husband, Roger, for 42 years. And I needed him with me for this journey. Some people were remembering how they felt when they lost their mom, dad, pet, etc. Soulmate grief is different. Yet, all forms of grief hurt and must be treated with care and caution. Some are strong-minded and can move on quickly. It still depends on the level of attachment and degree of love and the relationship. Many that are grieving are not as strong. What you see is not always the way it is with hurting people. I was the one that showed up positive and was crying and hurting away from everyone. If God can get me through grief and cancer at the same time, I know that he will and can get me through the fog of death. My soulmate was not with me which made me hurt so badly. However, God became my husband. God took care of me in ways I could not imagine. My children, sisters, brothers, friends, and co-workers rallied around me. Mr. Pearson and the administrative team of Sumter High School were so supportive and caring. I saw the hand of God in the total equation. God knew my past and blessed my present and gave me a bright future in my job before I retired. Others brought me organic foods, water, and healthy snacks, including my sisters sowing seeds on my trips to chemotherapy. My Christian friends comforted me with the word of God, visited me, and did their best to keep me encouraged as I battled grief and cancer. The blessings of the Lord began to manifest. Financially, God was sustaining me on one salary. I lost all of my husband's income and the Veterans Administration was fighting me on receiving my husband's military benefits. Abba Father, my husband was taking care of me, so I will never beg for bread. (Psalm 37:25)

They all were the workings of my Abba Father God who kept his promises to me. I saw the hand of God in the people he used to bless me. I had to seek and find the place where God was meeting me and that is when my entire mindset changed. No one could have an encounter with the Lord and remain the same. I felt different and I began to love wholeheartedly. I also saw the devil's hand in ones that came to discourage me, get into my business, and get me angry when I failed to do what they thought that I should do. They had no compassion for what I was going through. They came to upset me, use me, and to dump garbage from their foul hearts. Through prayer, they stopped bothering me and I was grateful. Not everyone that claims that they are on God's assignment is on God's assignment. They did not prevail. At my weakest point, God became my strength. On days that the chemo had me weak and sick, God strengthened my children especially my wonderful daughter, Renata, to step up and hold the house together. God also blessed my oldest son, Roger J.T., to move home to care for his mother along with my youngest son, Ricardo. My sisters and close friends visited frequently to check on me and lift my spirits as well. The spirit of God kept all my three children and my six grandchildren. They were so afraid of losing me after just losing their dad and granddad, Roger. God kept all of us. I saw fear in my baby's face. My Ricardo, that lived with me and spent each and every day with his dad was hurting immensely. My cancer remission was on the doctor's terms but to me, God has completely healed me. We walk by faith and not by sight according to 2 Corinthians 5:7. I told someone that God was such a showoff. He knew that I was going through the fog of grief and then He gave Satan permission to afflict me with cancer to show off His glory while grieving for only 4 months. He knows that I will forever praise Him and testify on His behalf about His goodness and power. God showed off "His glory."

The Cancer That I Was Diagnosed With

I was diagnosed with HER2-positive breast cancer. This is a type of breast cancer that tests positive for a protein called human epidermal growth factor receptor 2 (HER2). This protein promotes the growth of cancer cells. In other words, HER2 is a protein that tells cells to grow. In HER2+ breast cancer, the cancer cells have too much HER2, which leads to cancer growth. These cancer cells grow and divide faster than healthy cells, causing tumors to form. HER2+ breast cancer can spread to other parts of the body. This is known as HER2+ metastatic breast cancer.

I give thanks to my heavenly Father that I was diagnosed and treated promptly since the cancer had only spread to the lymph nodes. I endured six months of chemotherapy, lumpectomy surgery, six weeks of radiation, and continuous visits to the oncologist, surgeon, radiologist, primary doctor, and heart doctor. It appears that once cancer is diagnosed, the doctor's visits are "never-ending." Nevertheless, I praise my Lord and Savior Jesus Christ for the diagnosis of "Remission." I say total HEALING. This term is used until five years of being diagnosed as "Cancer-Free" is established. To continue my health, I am taking a hormone receptor that blocks estrogen.

In about 1 of every 5 breast cancers, the cancer cells have extra copies of the gene that makes the HER2 protein. HER2-positive breast cancers tend to be more aggressive than other types of breast cancer.

Treatments that specifically target HER2 are very effective. These treatments are so effective that the prognosis for HER2-positive breast cancer is quite good. In all and through all, God is to be praised. According to 2 Corinthians 1:4, God comforts us in all our troubles or afflictions so that we can comfort those who are in any affliction, with the comfort we are comforted by God.

Be comforted, be encouraged, but most of all, have no fear. "Faith and Fear" cannot live in the same house. Pray until you can walk in peace, faith, and love. Let the healing begin.

Practice Makes "IT" Better
Karen Owens Blanding

Practice can be used as a noun or a verb. I am using it as a verb. Practice, by definition, means *"perform an activity or a skill repeatedly or regularly in order to improve or maintain one's proficiency."* You will understand more about why this title fits this chapter as you read my story.

Here goes...

I was 44 years old in 2007 and life was good. I had married my high school sweetheart after losing contact for 10 years. We had three children. Just two years prior I had landed a "good" job with the federal government. Life was really good and I felt good too. My home was happy. My children were involved in band, sports, choir, church...you name it. I was serving on school committees, church committees, work committees, and Alpha Kappa Alpha Sorority, Inc. committees. We were a busy family just living life and BAM...I felt a little rock at the top of my right breast. Surely it wasn't cancer! I didn't smoke. I didn't drink much, maybe 3 times a year. I never worked in a factory or around chemicals. I ate healthily. I took vitamins. I even ate broccoli!

I kept this little rock to myself for a week or so and then I told my husband. He immediately encouraged me to get it checked out. I went to the GYN doctor, who referred me to the mammogram center. The mammogram was inconclusive so I was recommended for an ultrasound. I went for the ultrasound and the doctor confirmed that there was something there but I was told not to worry. It was just cysts filled with fluid. Fluid-filled cysts, huh? I can handle that. I asked what to do about this cyst and the doctor told me I could opt to do nothing and the fluid would likely dissolve and go away. Or, I could follow up with a surgeon and have the fluid analyzed.

I opted to do nothing. Why? I couldn't imagine the possibility of ME having breast cancer. Not at my age. Not with my health history. Not with my healthy habits. It was probably nothing. The mammogram was in February. The little rock in my breast didn't appear to be connected to any breast tissue. I could roll it around like a marble under some cover. I was so pleased with the good news of "no cancer" I did not follow the recommendation to do a monthly breast exam. Fast-forward to August. Six months had passed and my husband asked me if I was keeping up with my breast exams. I wasn't. I reluctantly agreed to do a self-check that evening just to satisfy him. I was certain there wasn't anything to be concerned about. To my surprise, this little rock wasn't just a little rock anymore. It had grown roots and appeared to be attached to breast tissue. OMG!! It didn't roll around like a marble anymore. It was dense and stuck. Now...I was concerned.

I reached out to the GYN, who had said the little rock was a fluid-filled cyst, and he referred me to a surgeon. I made an appointment with the surgeon to test the fluid. I arrived for my consultation with the surgeon alone. It had been six months since my mammogram. The surgeon received the film from six months ago but he wanted to get an up-to-date image to see if anything had changed. I have an inquiring mind, so I asked the doctor to let me see the ultrasound while he was doing it. I remembered how the fluid-filled cysts looked six months ago and it was like I was looking at the wrong image. It was NOTHING like six months before. The surgeon said the same thing. He was wondering if he had received the wrong image. We both were bewildered. This was supposed to be a quick and fast consultation. My appointment was taking a long time. The surgeon asked that I come back to do a biopsy. What he saw on the image did not appear to be fluid-filled.

I returned to the office, alone, on a Thursday for the biopsy. Being alone was my choice. I didn't have to be sedated. I received some numbing medicine through a needle and then a little piece of skin was plucked out of my breast to be sent to the lab. I was so sure it was going to be nothing and I didn't see a need to involve anyone else. The biopsy was done. The mass was so thick that it felt like a piece of concrete was stopping the needle. It would take 2 days to get the results, so I would have to wait through the weekend and get my results on Monday. There was nothing to do now but wait.

I WASN'T READY

I returned Monday to get the results. I was alone. Again, this was my choice. When I went to the window of the receptionist to check-in, I was asked if I was at the appointment by myself. I found that strange. I had never been asked that before. I replied that I was alone and the receptionist asked if I wanted to wait for a friend or family member to come. That was strange too. I said no. It came to my turn to be called to the back. As I walked through the door, the nurse also asked if I was alone. I said yes, and she also asked if I wanted to wait for someone to come. AGAIN, I said NO. Things still didn't click for me right away. The nurse proceeded to lead me to an area of the building that I didn't know existed. I turned a few corners and went down a couple of hallways and ended up in a room far, far away. The room had an office desk, two chairs, and a box of Kleenex. That was weird. Now I'm concerned. The doctor peeked in and saw me sitting alone and asked if I was waiting on someone to come. It was at this point, I concluded that it would be a good idea to call my husband since I was asked the same question three times.

The doctor offered to give me time to contact someone to be with me. I called my husband and he was in the office in 10 minutes. The doctor came in and delivered the news. I had cancer cells in my breast tissue and it had spread to two lymph nodes. Stage 2 Triple Negative Breast Cancer. In those six months of waiting, cancer had spread to my lymph nodes. Once the doctor said cancer, I didn't hear anything else for a minute. I'm so glad my husband was there to listen. I was coming back to reality. Then it hit me! That's why they all wanted me to have someone with me. They thought I was going to break down. They took me further back, behind all of the halls and curves, so I could cry out and not disturb the other waiting patients. My husband was devastated. I could see the pain in his face. He didn't know what to think or what to do. I was stunned and I don't believe I heard much after that. I learned that it's a good idea to have someone with you that can listen while you try to process everything. My husband and I both had people in our circle who did not survive their cancer diagnosis. Did this mean my days were numbered? Did this mean that I needed to say my goodbyes and get my business in order? What did this mean for me? For us? For our young sons? My mind was racing.

I NEEDED A PLAN

The surgeon went on to say that I needed to have surgery right away. He had an opening for Thursday. That was just three days away. My sons ranged in age from nine to thirteen. I had to get things arranged for them. I needed to wash clothes. Pay for their lunch in advance, get uniforms and game equipment organized....oh and work....I needed to reschedule appointments. There was so much to be done. I put everything and everybody before me and put the surgery off. I scheduled my surgery to take place a week later. My husband and I were driving separately, so I made my way to the car. I told my sister-in-law when I was going to receive my test results and she didn't give me a chance to call her. I had just pulled away from the hospital parking lot and my cell phone was ringing. I stared at it for a few rings; trying to decide what I was going to say. The phone rang for the 4th time and I answered. When she asked me what the doctor said, I couldn't get the words out. I could not get myself to say, "I have cancer". I began to sob quietly and she instantly knew. I needed to get home. My vision was blurred. I could hardly see the road to drive. I felt like I was losing control. I had to get myself together so I could at least get home safely. I told my sister-in-law that I needed to hang up and I would call her later. I took a slow ride home trying to pull myself together. I felt like people around me would pick up on my energy, so I needed to be "strong". This also meant that I had to continue to share my diagnosis with the loved ones in my life. Trying to say the word cancer for the first time was hard, but now I needed to say it over, and over, and over again. Each person wanted to hear the story about how it was found. I wasn't ready. **WOULD I EVER BE READY?**

If I could get a do-over, I would have followed up with the surgeon immediately, but there is no place for a do-over now. That moment in time is now history. I won't put off health questions anymore. When in doubt, I will check it. I had a few people that shared (in great detail) the horrible experiences and deaths of people they knew who had gone through cancer. I began to wonder about myself. Am I going to die THAT way? How long do I have to live? What will happen to my children? Husband? Parents? Should I be making funeral arrangements while I have the strength? Thoughts of death and trying to predict my journey to death began to consume me.

DECISION TO CHANGE

My mind was racing. I needed to quiet these thoughts down. Everything started to settle in. I arrived home and took a moment to reflect on my perfect life. I thought about being sick like other people I knew or had heard about. I rehearsed my death and tried to guess what it was going to look like to die at my age. I beat myself up for not doing my monthly breast exam. Would things be different if I had followed up earlier? It still would have been cancer, but it wouldn't have had a chance to spread. In the quiet of the night, it happened. I finally broke down. I cried until my shoulders were shaking and the tears were meeting under my chin and dripping onto my chest. I was a mess. Where was my faith? I had to stop this stinkin' thinkin'. I concluded that I was going to have to practice keeping God's word close to my heart and my mouth. I would have to turn my thoughts from negative to positive. I would have to practice positive thinking at all times. I would have to learn to practice putting my faith in front of my fears. This is when my "IT" became my FAITH. I remembered the "Serenity Prayer".

Prayer for Serenity

God, grant me the serenity
to accept the things I cannot change,
the courage to change the things I can,
and the wisdom to know the difference.
Living one day at a time,
enjoying one moment at a time;
accepting hardship as a pathway to peace;
taking, as Jesus did,
this sinful world as it is,
not as I would have it;
trusting that You will make all things right
if I surrender to Your will;

so that I may be reasonably happy in this life
and supremely happy with You forever in the next.
Amen.

By: Reinhold Niebuhr

The Serenity Prayer was the thing that kept me grounded. I had to practice doing some things on purpose, but first I had to determine what things I had total control over. The one thing I had absolute total control over would be the people that I allowed to speak into my life. "People" could be relatives, co-workers, friends, family, Sorors, neighbors, or even the good sisters at the church.

People should know better than to share horrible death stories, but they do not. Why in God's name would anybody with any ounce of compassion, choose to tell someone with a cancer diagnosis–cancer death stories?? I immediately put the "Serenity Prayer" into practice. "Courage to change the things I can."

People speaking negative energy over my life were dismissed without delay. I didn't make an announcement. I made myself unavailable. I practiced surrounding myself with positive energy and positive conversation. I changed the people I was around. I am not oblivious to the natural progression of life. The scripture tells us that no one knows the day nor the hour of the final moments on earth. I refuse to waste one moment of any day that God has gifted me operating as if I am dying.

I WILL LIVE

I will live until God has decided that I have done ALL that He has set out for me to do and I have touched ALL the lives He has anointed me to touch. I had to get myself together.

Tomorrow will come and it will be a new day. This new day would be the beginning of my new normal. Cancer and the mess that comes with a cancer diagnosis were now a part of my life. I couldn't change that. I did have the power to change how I thought about it. I made a conscious decision to trust the word of God. Practicing my "it"–FAITH.

I couldn't operate in fear. It was time for me and the Lord to get together. In the midst of my pity party, I began to realize that I had so much to thank God for. I had family and friends in my circle that I could count on. I had insurance. I actually had two medical plans. I had a loving, reliable, and responsible husband who had made a very comfortable life and home for our family. I had a reliable car. I had Jesus. I got busy preparing for surgery and my new normal after surgery and recovery while preparing my extended family to help manage the extracurricular activities of my three young sons. I wanted them to go to every practice, every game, every performance, and every PTA. I wanted to keep their lives as close to the same as possible.

MY NEW NORMAL

The week of my cancer diagnosis was a blur. I washed and ironed, packed, prayed, and prepared. My husband didn't talk much. I didn't either. We just did what was necessary to be done. We did it together. He was there. I can't begin to imagine this journey with anyone else. My husband has a quiet but strong presence that has a way of making you feel that there is nothing to worry about. That's what I needed.

The day of surgery went without any hiccups. I expected to spend the night. My husband was with me the entire time and was at my side as soon as he could be there after surgery. The anesthesia started to wear off and I began to get hungry. My meal came and I decided that I didn't want to lay flat in the bed to eat so I sat on the side of the bed with my feet dangling. My Pastor stopped by to visit and I could see the shocked look on her face. I got thrown off by her reaction and didn't know what to say to change the awkwardness of the moment. I wondered what she saw that resulted in such a stare.

After a brief moment of silence, she told me that she had visited many people after cancer surgery and I was the only person she had ever seen sitting on the side of the bed having dinner. Being able to witness that moment was a blessing for her. That moment spoke to me as well. I realized that I should not base my journey on any journey I had heard about. I needed to stop imagining my death and live my life to the fullest. God sent her to me to get the message that He was in control of my journey! And this was confirmation that I needed to stop imagining and visualizing my demise. I had verification that my journey would be designed by God and only God.

God did not promise me that I wouldn't have obstacles. His promise was that He would be with me. Practicing my faith made my cancer journey better. The reality is that everyone living has to die. None of us know the day, the week, the hour, or how. It's all in God's time, but for now, I am living this day that the Lord has made, I will rejoice and be glad in it; taking one day at a time.

I arrived at the hospital with both breasts. I left the hospital with one breast and a row of staples. This was my first real challenge in accepting the things I could not change. I stood in the mirror looking at myself and didn't know what to think. That was an ugly sight for me to behold, so I was pretty sure my husband didn't want to see my body like that. I needed to figure out how I could keep this shielded from him. I was supposed to have received a pair of foam prostheses when I left the hospital. I didn't get them. This was my first time going through a mastectomy. I didn't know to ask for them. I got dressed and the flat chest stuck out like a sore thumb. How could my husband stand to look at me when I couldn't stand to look at myself? I struggled with body changes. I walked around pretending and dodging my husband. I tried to keep my distance from him. I wanted to leave the house and go somewhere…anywhere. Where was I going to go with one breast? I was ashamed and I didn't have the right clothes. My oldest son had a band concert at his middle school and I wanted to attend. I put on my husband's jean jacket, which was oversized, and prayed that people wouldn't notice the asymmetry as I took my seat in the car on the way to the band concert. I attended that concert with one breast and guess what?? Nobody noticed.

ACCEPTING HELP

This seems to be a good place to insert the importance of having a support system/caregivers. Sickness can happen to anyone. It doesn't matter how much money you have, how many degrees you have, how many cars you drive, or how independent you think you are. When cancer or any sickness comes upon you, you need a support system. You need people. It is good for the soul to know that you are not in the fight alone. My family was awesome. My husband, Bernard Blanding stepped right in to cook, clean, wash clothes, or do anything else he could do. I reached out to him to reflect on his experience as a caregiver to get his viewpoint on anything he felt a caregiver should know. He said it's important for the caregiver to know that once sickness raises its ugly head, the caregiver must immediately realize that it's all about the person who is going through the illness. Things will no longer be what you are used to. The hardest part is when the rock of the home is unable to take care of all the things the family has become accustomed to. He also said being a caregiver means there is no room for feeling like you can't do something because you have never done it before. You have to face some things head-on to get more practice at doing what you are not used to. Get comfortable being uncomfortable. Practicing "it" makes it better. You might not like it. It may not be easy. You might make some mistakes and mess a few things up, but IT will get better. Will you make a mistake? Yes. Will you forget the Gatorade for practice? Lunch money? Or miss the barbershop? Yes, but tomorrow will come and it will be another chance to be better than yesterday. Keep practicing. In the midst of all of that, we cannot be hesitant about accepting help. I had a moment where I needed help practicing one of my "its". Accepting help didn't come naturally to me. I was determined to be as self-sufficient as I could. I needed help bathing…but I wouldn't ask. I needed help dressing…but I wouldn't ask. I was climbing on footstools and doing all sorts of hazardous things, trying to be independent. In my mind, I thought I was being helpful to my family by doing some things on my own, and then one day I had the notion to go to a caregiver's support group at the cancer center. God directed me there. I had no business there. I was the patient, NOT the caregiver. There was a gentleman there that was very transparent. He explained to the group how awful cancer had been to his dear wife. He said that he had always been able to fix things to make them better for her but with cancer, his hands were tied and he felt helpless. If she had a taste for a certain flavor of ice cream and it was two in the morning, he wanted her to ask him to go get it and he would jump in the car to bring that ice cream back as fast as he could if having ice cream made things better for her. In other words, he welcomed the invitation to be helpful because that's all he could do. I shared the story with my husband and he agreed with the gentleman. The moral of this story is… Let your caregivers care. They want to be there for you.

I have a dear friend, who came into my life when my baby boy was attending the daycare where she was working. I am not sure when we became friends, but we did and nobody but the good Lord above could have known how instrumental she would be during my breast cancer journey. Not only was she there, but she wanted to be there. She never made me feel like she was doing anything because she felt obligated. It was in her nature to be caring and she was. Her presence in my life made the new normal after cancer bearable for me and especially for my young sons. She was a surrogate grandmother, taxi driver, chef, and friend. I am forever grateful for her presence in our lives.

BACK TO WORK

It came time for me to return to work, and I didn't have the right stuff to wear. I still had not been made aware of the breast forms that should have been given to me immediately after surgery or shortly afterward, and I was at a loss for what to do. There I stood, staring at myself in the mirror, disgusted by what I saw. The missing breast was quite noticeable, and I was horrified by what I was looking at with or without clothes on. I managed to put together a few outfits with jackets and pressed my way. I did this for a few days and it happened again. Stinkin' thinkin'. I found myself sitting on the side of the bed crying. I was feeling down and sorry for myself. None of my shirts fit properly. They were all cut to low. I didn't like the jackets. Nothing hung right. Nothing matched. I felt ugly and ashamed. My husband snuck up on me and caught me crying. I never wanted him to seem weak so I made it a point to keep tears to myself. God said no to lonely tears this time. Of course, my husband asked what was wrong, and as I tried to speak between heavy breaths and sobs, I somehow managed to babble enough that he was able to figure out what the problem was. He gently wrapped his arms around me and held me so close and whispered that he would choose me over my breast any day of the week. That made me smile. (But where was my faith?) I started to

58

clean myself up but was still not feeling so good about my wardrobe. My husband had a solution that was so simple. Let's go shopping. I reflected back to the Serenity prayer which it says to change the things that you can. It took me by surprise how easy I slipped into this place of pity when I had so much to thank God for. My husband reminded me that we did not have to decide between buying clothes and buying medicine. I must say that my dear husband was a wonderful provider. He made a lot of good decisions along the way that allowed us to be okay financially. He told me that he has never said to me that I could not buy what I needed and he wasn't going to start. He told me to go shopping and buy some things that fit the way I wanted them.

I reflected back on my cry and I had to ask myself...you mean to tell me, it was that simple? How did I get to this moment? I stopped practicing my faith walk. I stumbled into that place of fear for a split second. That's the advantage of keeping positive people in your life. They know how to speak life and prosperity over you. I could have thought myself into a deep depression about something as simple as clothes. My wardrobe was a big deal to me, yet, my husband made it simple. Look at how God worked through him. We went shopping.

Chemo and radiation were recommended for my treatment plan. I had heard so many horror stories about the side effects of chemo and I wanted to be proactive in trying to be as healthy as possible while getting treatment. My children were participating in quite a few activities and I wanted to be well and in attendance.

CHOOSING CTCA

I went to my first consultation. The oncologist had a standard treatment plan for everyone with breast cancer. That visit didn't feel right to me. I felt like I was just another cancer patient and she didn't care much about me as an individual. I felt that she was just checking a box. I asked the oncologist if there were any vitamins or regimens she could recommend that would help me stay well. She told me that if I had extreme diarrhea or vomiting to let her know. I explained that I wanted to keep those two things at bay as much as I could, so I explained more by asking again if there was something I could do to be proactive. She told me to just let her know when or if it was extreme, and she would prescribe something if I needed anything. That was disappointing. I began to search for a second opinion. I found a second oncologist. They also had a standard way of treating breast cancer. I figured that this must be how it is everywhere, so I asked the nurse if she could tell me things I could do that would help me to not be sick. She told me to contact them before I took anything. That response puzzled me. Their practice was open for twenty-two years, they should have had a list of things to share with me. That was disappointing as well. Neither of those experiences settled well with me. I didn't want to go to treatment with either one of them. My husband supported my decision and wanted me to be comfortable with my choice of care. I tried to call both doctors to ask questions. Each time I was sent to voicemail and waited all day for a callback. I called the next day and spoke to a nurse. I waited all day for a callback. I called the third day and got a different nurse. She wasn't aware of my call and I had to share my concern again. I waited again…all day for a callback. This was aggravating. My husband was working a job where he went to work at midnight. He didn't want me to be home without assistance, so he organized a system for a family member or friend to stay with me overnight. There are always little blessings in unfortunate situations. My little blessing was having my father as a caregiver. My dad was always too busy, but while I was recovering, he would spend some nights with me. We would reminisce and watch TV. Breast cancer allowed me to have some precious moments with my father that we would have been too busy to have. I thank God for having that. My father and I were watching TV at about 3 AM and a commercial for the Cancer Treatment Centers of America (CTCA) came on. My dad suggested that I try CTCA. At the time of my diagnosis, the center for me would be in Zion, Illinois, or Philadelphia, Pennsylvania. The Atlanta, Georgia facility wasn't built yet. South Carolina didn't have the option for CTCA. Illinois and Pennsylvania were too far to travel so I let CTCA leave my mind. My dad saw the commercial again and wrote down the number. You have to have known my father to know how serious this was for him to take the time to find paper and pen to write down a number. I felt like it was God's way of directing my path, so I called the 800 number and I was sent to the voicemail of a case manager. I had become used to doctor's offices not returning calls, but I left a message anyway and checked the box of making the call so I could tell my father that I had made the call and my words would be true. Low and behold a case manager called me back in less than an hour. That was different for me and I liked that a lot. I had a brief conversation to ask a few questions to share the answers with my family and also gave my contact information. I had asked God to order my steps, but surely He wasn't leading me to CTCA in Zion, Illinois, which was almost 900 miles from my home. I had a few more questions and decided to call again two days later. This time a different person answered the phone. To my surprise, she was aware of my previous calls and asked me if I had gotten the answer to my previous questions. She reviewed what was discussed on my previous call, and she assisted me with getting answers to my new questions. This was nothing like any of my experiences with the local doctors. Do you remember reading where I called multiple times without a return call? Not to mention having to repeat myself with each callback?

I asked the same question as I had done with the other oncology clinics. Are there medications or vitamins to take to help me be healthy while going through treatment? She informed me that they had a naturopathic doctor, and their facility valued the importance of traditional medicines and natural medicines. WOW!!! She went on to say they would consider the results of my labs, type of cancer, and a few other things to determine what vitamin regimen and treatment would work best for me. I was pleasantly surprised by CTCA. I wanted to go there even though it was miles and miles away. I had to go there. They seemed to care about me as an individual. They didn't have a cookie-cutter treatment plan. And they returned phone calls. I wanted to be a patient there so bad. I talked it over with my husband and parents and they supported my decision. They couldn't understand it, but they supported it. I moved forward to schedule a flight for a third opinion at the CTCA in Zion, Illinois. It's hard for many to understand why I was willing to travel from SC to Illinois for treatment. It means a lot to be made to feel like you matter and I felt like I mattered to them. I was someone's mom, sister, daughter, wife, or auntie, and not just another cancer diagnosis. I felt like I was seen and not just a box to check off. I felt like family. We scheduled our trip to the "Windy City" and were on the way within a week. I found out after I arrived that CTCA had a philosophy to treat each patient as if they were your mother. How amazing is that? I was confident that I had chosen the right place.

My breast cancer diagnosis was in 2007 with Dr. Dennis Citrin as my oncologist at CTCA in Zion, IL. He was so gentle and kind. He spent more than 30 minutes with my husband and me, explaining the type of cancer I had, the stage, treatment plan, chemo side effects, etc. He literally drew a picture when I needed further explanation. Dr. Citrin noticed my make-shift outfit to camouflage my breast and asked me if I had received breast forms, mastectomy camisole, etc. I had not. He referred me to the "Look Good Feel Better" department. The ladies there helped me get fitted for the breast form. I was able to take my jacket off for the first time in months. I felt refreshed. Needless to say, we decided to take the trip to Zion, IL every 21 days for chemotherapy treatment. We were committed. We later came to realize the Cancer Treatment Centers of America has what they call the "Mother Standard of Care". In other words, you are treated the way they would like your mother to be treated. That explained the callback and attention to detail. It sealed the deal for me and my family.

HAIR LOSS

I received my treatment schedule. I was keenly aware that there was a good possibility that I was going to lose my hair. I took a bold move and cut my hair to about 2 inches thinking the shock of losing so much hair would be lessened, and I wanted to feel like I was in control. I had heard all the horror stories about people waking up and finding clumps of hair on the pillow; an entire wad of hair on a roller on the pillow, going through their routine of combing or brushing their hair to find the entire section of hair has been pulled out or even put shampoo on their hair to watch it drop to the drain in large patches. I didn't want to experience that, so cutting my hair was my way of coping and taking control. I began chemotherapy, and every day I would take a pinch of hair at the nape of my neck and pull it to see if it was still hanging on. I did this every day. Somewhere about three weeks after my first treatment, I reached back to take a pinch of hair and whatever I was holding between my fingers came out. It's crazy how I expected it every day, but hoped it wouldn't happen and then celebrated when it was still there. Each day I felt it was a chance that I could be in the small percentage of people who didn't lose their hair. I stood looking at the clump of hair between my fingers, not knowing what to do. I wasn't sure what I was feeling, but today was surely a different feeling from yesterday. My hair had lost its grip from the root. My husband, my rock, stepped in with the clippers. He reminded me that we made a decision to be in control of cancer and we couldn't stop now. Instead of allowing cancer to remove my hair at its convenience, I sat in front of the bathroom mirror and my husband took control and shaved my head. UUUUGGGHHHH. I was bald. Not a wig or hat in sight. I am usually pretty good at planning ahead, but for some reason, being proactive about getting a wig didn't cross my mind. If I could do that moment over, I would have taken my time to buy a good wig before losing my hair.

Instead of having a good plan, I went out in a panic trying to get a wig. I had never worn a wig, so my wig experience was interesting. I wasn't bold about my bald head and knew nothing about the wig selection process. I went to the first store and learned that I had to try the wig on in the back aisle of the store, rather than in a private room. You guessed it. I had to display my bald head to whoever was around each time. That was humiliating to me. I wasn't going to keep doing that. My solution was to just buy wigs and take them home to try them out. I wasted quite a bit of money because once I purchased the wigs, I couldn't take them back. I purchased quite a few wigs that I didn't like. I shouldn't say the money was wasted. I ended up donating the wigs to a local cancer foundation that gave wigs to those who didn't have insurance. I never quite learned how to put the wigs on straight so they were often a tiny bit off-center or pulled too far up or too far back. That is funny to me now, but back then it was an awful time.

LOOKING ON THE BRIGHT SIDE

There were quite a few of life's lessons during my breast cancer journey. I didn't know anything about wigs, so every day with wigs was an adventure. Imagine how shocked I was to learn that you shouldn't bake bread with your synthetic wig on because the heat melts the ends together. Who knew?? I had such a time with my search for wigs that I ended up with a small collection. I decided that I would have fun with the wigs. Why couldn't I treat my wigs as an accessory? I could get wigs in different colors and lengths. Right? I went to my son's middle school one day and I wore a short wig. I went to the school a few weeks later and wore a long wig. Something came up and I had to go by the school again and I happened to mention that I was planning a trip to see the teacher. My son pulled me to the side and told me to please make up my mind which head of hair I was going to wear, so I could wear the same one to his school. That was hilarious to me. I didn't think they paid attention to that type of thing.

A sweet moment for me and my family was when my husband and 3 sons staged a candlelight dinner for me. It was a little odd because the house was dark. They sat me at the table and fumbled around for something to light the candle. Once the candle was lit, I saw my husband first in the flicker of light. He had shaved his head!! OMG...the next candle was lit and what was the reveal? The boys had shaved their heads to go through the bald phase of cancer with me. I was overwhelmed and I cried. My husband had a nice head of wavy hair that he swooped up like Peabo Bryson. I am sure that was a sacrifice to cut off his curly locks. My sons were at the age where peer opinion mattered and they still did that for and with me. I would never be able to express how deeply my heart melted when I saw them all so proud to stand with me. It turned out that my husband had an element of sexy that was hidden behind his head of hair. His bald head was quite appealing. He never went back.

B to D CUP

Initially, I wanted to have reconstruction surgery so I looked into breast implants. I had been a B cup all my life and decided to have a little fun. I told the surgeon that I wanted to go to a D cup. That was going to be exciting for me. The procedure involved putting in temporary implants and injecting fluid/saline into my breast tissue to stretch the skin. It put a new meaning to no pain, no gain. My skin was tight and didn't give easily. I had planned a five-day cruise with the family that was scheduled around the implant visits. I began to run a fever seven days before we were scheduled to go. I went to the emergency room to find out I had developed an infection at the implant site. I always carry a large purse that has everything, from a screwdriver and flashlight to Tylenol and Kleenex. Not today. I traveled to the emergency room with a pouch. There was nothing in it but my identification and insurance cards. I was admitted to the hospital. The doctor tried to treat the infection without removing the implant. And that didn't work. My temperature was being monitored. It kept going up to 103. I wanted to dupe the system by taking Tylenol when the medical staff wasn't looking, so I could keep the fever down. So I asked my husband to bring my big purse. He wouldn't do it. That's crazy to me now because I would have been on a cruise full of infection. They say the Lord takes care of babies and fools, and He took care of me by keeping me away from my personal bottle of Tylenol. I would have been on my way to a five-day boat cruise if I could have had it my way. I was told that if my temperature spiked once more I would be in surgery the next day, which would also be the same day we were scheduled to be on the cruise. My temperature spiked and my mother and father agreed to accompany our 3 sons on the cruise while my husband stayed back to be with me during surgery. That experience helped me to decide to let the D cup go. I wanted to get back to my life and the process for the implants proved to be a hindrance to my healing speed. The doctor said the shelf life of the implant could be 17-20 years. Who needs perky breasts at 65??? Would I want to be going through surgery at 65 years old to remove or replace implants?? I decided I didn't and opted to use breast forms. Breast forms came in a D cup as well, so all was not lost. I could still go for a larger look. I tried the D cup and they were heavy. No wonder I wasn't blessed with large breasts. I couldn't handle it. I traded in my D cup for a C cup, which was much more comfortable, and I never looked back.

My husband was great about the entire process. He told me that he would support any decision I made but asked that I not get implants because I felt like he wanted them. Initially, I thought he was telling me what I wanted to hear, but he truly meant it. I took him at his word and let go of the possibility of implants. The kind of love my husband demonstrates to me is not what is common. I have met one or two couples whose relationship didn't make it through this body transformation. Losing a breast or two was too much of a negative change for their significant others. I ended up having a double mastectomy, with my husband's support, and I would often get a confidence boost from the lyrics of a song by India Arie entitled "*I Am Not My Hair*". I am the soul that lives within. I am the prize. If breasts, or lack of breasts, affect how I am seen, it is the other person's loss. Not mine. Period. I am grateful for my husband. We made it through the transformation. He appreciated my soul.

CHALLENGING MYSELF

I made the best of my time getting chemo. CTCA allowed me to use a laptop while I sat for four to eight hours, receiving the chemo infusion. I made the best of it and registered for a class. I completed a three-hour online course while having chemotherapy. Can you believe that? I concluded that I was going to live each day like I had the gift of tomorrow. I was only going to leave this earthly place when the Lord God saw fit and not before. I would not waste the day the Lord had given me refusing to live. I kept this attitude throughout my journey of recovery and healing. Things were back to normal again. I did not have to take a chemo pill. I continued to travel to CTCA in Zion, Illinois for check-ups. I started out going every three weeks. I progressed to every three months; then every six months, and finally once a year! That was refreshing. My husband and I would make the best of the trips to Illinois. We would often take a walk to the movie theater or catch the train to the zoo. We even visited the jelly belly jelly bean factory to see just how jelly beans were made. We purposely searched for things to do that would make our trips to the cancer center more than just a doctor's visit. We made memories.

My trips to CTCA, Zion Illinois began in 2007 and they still continue to this day, but it's not to keep a check on my breast health anymore. I was diagnosed with Multiple Myeloma in June of 2018. Multiple Myeloma is a blood cancer that is a cousin to Leukemia. I practiced my faith through the second diagnosis of cancer, treatment, and recovery process just as I did the first time. The breast cancer journey was a breeze compared to Multiple myeloma. Perhaps I will write about that experience another time. Until then, I will diligently work to continue to be an example of God's healing, grace, and mercy as I am a living testimony.

KAREN'S DAILY DECLARATION OF HEALING

I am totally healed. It is God's desire that I be healed and victorious. I declare that on this day I am walking in God's prosperity and His blessings are on every aspect of my life. I am spiritually well and no weapon formed against me shall prosper. I am totally healed through faith, medicine, and mindset. **GOD IS A HEALER.**

Playlist for Lyrical uplift

JEFFREY LAMPKIN ~ Keep Holding On
INDIA ARIE ~ I Am Not My Hair
DONALD LAWRENCE & THE TRI-CITY SINGERS ~ Encourage Yourself
ANTHONY BROWN & GROUP therAPy ~ Trust in You
MISSISSIPPI MASS CHOIR ~ When I Rose
ANTHONY BROWN & GROUP therAPy ~ This Week

HYMNAL ~ God Will Take Care of You
HELEN MILLER ~ I Won't Let You Fall
HEZEKIA WALKER ~ Better
VASHAWN MITCHELL ~ Turning Around
KURT CARR ~ I've Seen Him Do It
J.J. HAIRSTON ~ After This
LUTHER BARNES ~ You Keep On Blessing Me
WILLIAMS BROTHERS ~ Living Testimony
HEZEKIAH WALKER ~ Jesus is My Help
CHARLES JENKINS & FELLOWSHIP CHICAGO ~ I Will Live

The Diagnosis: My love, My Faith, My Healing
Kathy N. Bellamy

It all started in late November of 2019. I had my mammogram scheduled as I do yearly. It was a cool crisp November morning on the day of the appointment. The appointment went well! Afterward, I went on to work to go about my day as usual. I expected the results within the week, which was normal. This time I received a call to come back in for a repeat mammogram because of an abnormality that didn't show up in the years before. I had a breast MRI and an ultrasound on December 27, 2019. I received the results and was referred to a surgeon to do a breast biopsy. During the biopsy, a biopsy clip was placed in the breast so that if needed, the area would be marked. The biopsy showed the calcification of cells in the breast. After speaking to the surgeon and discussing the results, he recommended a lumpectomy. A lumpectomy is a surgical procedure where the cancerous tumor and an area of tissue surrounding it are removed. It also leaves the breast deformed or abnormally shaped. I could live with that as long as I still had life. The procedure was scheduled for 1/16/2020. Well, upon having the lumpectomy and meeting with the surgeon to discuss the results. He stated that 4 sides of the specimen were clean (no findings) but 2 sides were questionable–pre-cancerous cells. The doctor stated he could do another lumpectomy but could not guarantee that he would be able to reach all of the areas or completely take care of what they had discovered. I had other areas of calcification. He told me I had Ductal Carcinoma In Situ (DCIS) which is cancer inside the ducts of the breast that has not grown through the wall of the duct into the surrounding tissues. Sometimes referred to as a pre-cancer. He stated because I had multiple affected areas, he would recommend a mastectomy. He did not recommend doing multiple lumpectomies because there would not be much breast tissue left.

I was devastated. How could I go from a healthy woman who went in for a routine mammogram and get to this point? He went on to state, that some people because the findings were precancerous, they opt not to have anything else done. He told me my options. I could wait and have another mammogram in 6 months. In thinking back, I did not want to wait 6 months, that would have been nerve-wracking. I remember the doctor stating you all are so calm and seem to be taking this news quite well. Little did he know we were in a state of shock and disbelief. Mark and I needed to discuss our options and just wrap our minds around this piece of information. We were given a big book that contained lots of valuable information. My surgeon was so patient and kind. Answering my questions, addressing my concerns. He made himself available on the weekends. He accepted our calls at night or whenever we needed to talk. That is not often the case with a doctor. I appreciated his bedside manner. After we had some time to discuss the situation, we met with the surgeon again and asked to have a second opinion. I was referred to a breast surgeon oncologist at MUSC in Charleston Hollings Cancer Treatment Center.

I had my first appointment there on January 30, 2020. This was the 1st of many trips to Charleston. There was so much uncertainty, so many questions. At that first appointment, we met with the nurse navigator who went over basic information, telling us about what she does and any resources she could offer us. We then met with the breast surgeon oncologist. She also wanted to do her own tests. This led to breast MRIs, breast ultrasounds, biopsies, lab work, etc. From the start of this, I had been praying so hard. I wondered if God heard my prayer. I know he was listening because he saw me thru. By the way, if you need to have a breast MRI done and you are claustrophobic, then definitely ask for something to help you relax. During a breast MRI you will be laying face down to go in the MRI machine and lay there still for however long the procedure takes. Imagine so many tests to be done. Meetings with the medical teams. Traveling early mornings and staying all day, having multiple appointments a day or several times a week. Not knowing when you will get a phone call to come back in for some other test or the test results are inconclusive. As this process continued, we had no idea where this would lead us. One test led to another. Lab work was completed during each visit. My veins didn't always cooperate, which meant getting stuck multiple times. Drinking plenty of water before your visit is supposed to help, but my bladder did not always want to wait for the duration of the trip. Yes, people will say I wouldn't let them stick me like that. Sure, anyone could say that when they're not the one needing the medical treatment. Thankfully the nurses had ways of solving the issue. I appreciate everything they did to lessen the times I would have to be stuck. The appointments kept coming.

During this time, I would try to work as much as possible, some days working half a day, other days not working at all because of the timing of the appointments. I'm thankful to have had a good supervisor who showed compassion and empathy because there were days when I wouldn't be able to give a full 24 hours notice. At the time I was the only person working in my assigned area. Therefore, someone else would have to fill in for me, I felt bad for having to be out of work so often, but my health was a priority. Everything was happening so fast. So much information was given. It seems like there wasn't time enough to process it all. After meeting with the breast surgeon oncologist and completing all the tests that were ordered by her, we met to discuss them all. We were shown the results, she pointed out on the mammogram and MRIs where the area of concern was. There were multiple spots. She agreed with the previous doctor regarding the mastectomy. I was just praying that the 2nd opinion would have been different.

Somewhere during all of this, I started noticing a nipple discharge. I immediately started thinking this can't be good. The color was reddish-brown. It is not normal to have a discharge unless you are nursing. Well, I didn't have a baby so there was no nursing. I wasn't ready to accept the loss of a breast. Again, being told because of the amount of calcification of cells, another lumpectomy would not be recommended. She also did not recommend waiting six months for another mammogram. While being at that appointment, she made a referral to see a plastic surgeon who would discuss all the options of reconstruction. In the meantime, I was scheduled for 2 biopsies that would be performed on the same day, so I would not have to be in the hospital on two different days. That was a lot of information to take in. While riding home I kept replaying over and over the decision, I would need to make. I prayed for clarity and asked God to be with me and guide me in making a decision. Mark remained supportive by being a great listener while I bounced my thoughts and ideas off of him. I asked his opinion, sometimes I don't think he knew what to say. He was dealing with as much as I was. I knew it was a lot for him to deal with as a spouse not knowing how it would affect him as a caretaker/support person. So many things ran through my mind. Not only dealing with the prospect of having cancer but also losing a part of my body. Of course, I wanted to live and be healthy. The human side of me was thinking about the physical side. I didn't know how I would look. Would my husband still love me or want to be with me as a woman? This was not something I was ready to deal with, but I knew a decision had to be made that would change my life forever. To some people, it may be just a matter of having surgery and moving on. Well for me, even though I knew there were options after surgery it still was not one I was ready to make. All the while I continued to pray and ask God for guidance. I cried and I prayed–petitioning God. I wanted clarity. I wanted peace. I just didn't know what to do. We sought spiritual guidance and asked for prayers. So on Wednesday, February 12, 2020, two biopsies were performed on the left side in two different areas of the breast. I went home praying for the best knowing; there was nothing else to be done but pray and wait. Friday, February 14, 2020, while at work I received a telephone call from the breast surgeon oncologist. She called to tell me the biopsy results were back, and it was indeed cancer. I was heartbroken. I knew it could be a possibility, but it still hit hard. She stated she did not want me to wait all weekend to hear about the results. I couldn't cry, I was numb. Valentine's Day will never be the same. I had been in touch with a friend during this time of waiting. I called her because she had been waiting and praying with me. She was so encouraging and asked if I needed someone to take me home. She stated her husband could take me home. She was not driving at the time. I told her I could drive home. I told my supervisor I had to leave. My husband was home when I got there. He knew something wasn't right by the look on my face. I told him I got the test results back. He was hurt. We cried together. When we could get ourselves together, I could tell him about the appointment the next week with the breast surgeon oncologist. We thought about not attending the conference that weekend, but my friend encouraged us to go and get away from the house. We needed to take just a little time away. I wasn't registered for the conference but I was able to use the time to be in the room, just me and God. I prayed and cried and prayed and cried some more. I made a few phone calls to my family. Some prayed with me. Some gave encouraging words. I tried to relax and enjoy some quiet time. I tried sleeping but my thoughts kept me from having a restful sleep. I kept pondering what was going to happen to me. I didn't want to die. I wondered, Lord why me? After praying, crying, and reading scriptures, I finally got myself together. I said Lord it is me and you. I know that this did not come as a surprise to you. I need you Lord to help me through this situation. Lord, you know the end before the beginning. I was able to relax some, after all, I knew God was still in charge. The weekend passed so quickly and we were back home to face reality.

We met with the breast surgeon, oncologist. She showed us the cancerous areas. I was diagnosed with stage 2b. I was Her2 positive, as I was told it was an aggressive type of cancer. It was hormone-induced. She stated I would need chemo, surgery, and then afterward radiation. She discussed in more detail the type of cancer I had and why it was important to get the treatment needed. She went on to explain that I would be referred to an oncologist who would explain how chemo works. The oncologist would determine the number of chemo treatments that would be needed. Also, I would meet the nurse navigator. I am sitting in her office just thinking this can not be happening. A referral was made to the oncologist in Florence. Within a couple of days, I received an appointment with the oncologist. Of course, going to the oncologist, I did not know what to expect.

There was a team of people waiting for me. Each person had a different role to play in my care. I was evaluated and examined. The oncologist was firm and direct. He explained the type of cancer I was diagnosed with is one that could grow fast. He wanted to begin treatment as soon as possible. I would be scheduled for 6 chemo treatments. He stated since I was diagnosed with an aggressive form of cancer, he would treat it aggressively. Meaning I may have many sick days. The treatment days would be long. The side effects would vary from one treatment to the other. I would be scheduled for treatment every 21 days. On that day, I also met with the nurse navigator. She was pleasant and welcoming. She offered advice on what to expect over the next several months. She made it known that we could contact her at any time with questions and concerns. She advised us to reach out to her if we had trouble with appointments or referrals. She was also the leader of the support group. She invited us to our first support group meeting that was being held within the week. We went home with our minds loaded with so much information. In the meantime, we were trying to continue with our daily routines.

We tried to be as positive as possible. Still praying and trusting God. I think I was a bucket of water. I didn't feel very strong. I wanted to talk to friends, or at least people who I thought were friends. I mentioned to someone that I thought "so and so" would have reached out to me. The reply was, "you kept things to yourself, and no one knew what was going on", so they didn't know what to say. I really did not say anymore but I thought to myself would someone really need to know what is going on with me to reach out to me. A simple I'm thinking of you, is there anything I can do or something encouraging would have been just fine. Maybe I was in my feelings, but it did hurt to hear.

Moving on, I prayed and asked God to show me who to speak to about my situation. After all, the human side of me wanted to have someone to confide in from time to time. After the appointment with the oncologist, we met with the surgeon to schedule a date to have the port put in. It would be an outpatient surgery. Lab work and an echocardiogram were scheduled. Pre registration had to be done and of course, I had to be made aware of my financial obligation before the surgery. After the echocardiogram was completed, the tech asked if she could say a prayer on my behalf. The day of the surgery came, while prepping for the surgery I encountered a very nice young lady who was the nurse. She was friendly and kind. She talked of her mother and grandmother who both experienced breast cancer. They both had different experiences. She was wise beyond her years. She asked if she could pray with me, and I said yes. I was asked if I was willing to have the chaplain come speak with me, and I agreed. God was sending people to me who I didn't know I needed. I thanked him daily. The procedure went well. My next appointment was back with the oncologist to set up the start date of my 1st chemo treatment. Even though there were some hiccups with the insurance approving some of the medication needed, we kept trying. Between the nurse practitioner and nurse navigator making phone calls and following up with the insurance company, the medication for chemo was finally approved. On my last day at work before my 1st treatment, my supervisor met me at the hair store to help me pick out a wig. I didn't know how soon it would be before I lost my hair. I'm thankful I had her support in that endeavor; a wig was purchased.

My 1st chemo treatment was scheduled for March 12, 2020. Meanwhile, the world was experiencing this disease called Covid-19: Coronavirus. It was widespread; making so many people sick all over the world. People were getting sick suddenly and it was spreading quickly. At the time, it was not known how it was spreading but it was definitely contagious. Everyone was told to wear a facemask for protection. The day arrived for my 1st treatment. We had to be at the hospital at 7:30 am. I was nervous and scared. I prayed all the way there. All I could do was lean on God. The song, "Jesus said you can lean on me I won't let you fall," came to mind. Since singing is not my talent, I hummed as much of it as I could. Mark was right there by my side.

At the hospital, because of all the sickness with the coronavirus, we had to go through special procedures for registration. Security at the hospital had to call registration to confirm that I was scheduled to be there. Once my appointment was confirmed, someone from security escorted us to the registration area. I got registered and was sent to the waiting area for lab work. Labs were drawn to make sure all of my blood levels were what they needed to be so that chemo could be administered. After labs were drawn, I was sent upstairs to the chemo floor. As early as it was, there were quite a few people already being treated. All of this was so foreign to me. They took my vitals and got my weight. All of this was needed so that it could be tracked from one treatment to the other. The oncology nurse introduced herself and explained how things should go for the day. In the meantime, I had to wait on the lab results to come back before treatment could begin. After waiting for a while my lab work came back and treatment began. I wasn't ready for the big stick to access my port. After that, it was pretty much smooth sailing. It started with fluids, my pre-meds, nausea & allergy meds, etc. Some bags were larger than others. I was able to take a short nap in between the meds. With all of this going in, along with all the water I had been drinking, it was time to go to the bathroom. That meant unplugging the IV pole and pushing it to the bathroom. It was awkward at first but I got used to it since I would have to go so many times. Pretty soon lunch was served and treatment continued. By the end of the day, I was exhausted. When it was finally time to go home, the nurse told me I would have to take a shot the next day that would help build up my blood cells. In the past, a patient would have to go back to the doctor's office the next day to receive the injection. Now patients are given a body injector called Neulasta Onpro that's placed on the abdomen or back of the arm. I chose to have mine placed on my abdomen. Once it is placed on the body, it will count down a few seconds then the needle injects itself into your body. It's a quick sting. The medicine is not injected until the next day. I was told to look for the little green light that should be blinking throughout the next day until the time for the medication to be administered. When it was time the next day, I should listen for the beep then the medication would be injected. Once injected I had to check to make sure there was no liquid or wet spots around the area. I needed to be sure all the medication went in, and that the needle was still in place. This medication would help to replenish white blood cells that could be lowered upon having chemo treatment. Before leaving the hospital, the nurse told me things to look out for such things as diarrhea, constipation, nausea, vomiting, pain, and lack of appetite. She reminded me to drink plenty of fluids at all times. The oncologist asked me to monitor my temperature and to report it to the office if it went above 99.9. A high temperature could mean an infection somewhere in the body. I was advised to not use a razor on my body. I was told I should refrain from getting manicures and pedicures while receiving chemo treatment because of nicks or cuts that could occur. It was about 4 pm when we could finally leave for the day. Thank God one treatment was behind me. We made it home and I was finally able to lay down and rest. I think I was too hyped up to sleep right away but sleep finally came. Mark was tired as well. I think he was mentally tired trying to be strong for me. The next day came and so did diarrhea. I was able to eat and drink. Everything stayed down for a while. I thought the day went well. That evening the medication was injected into my abdomen and I took the patch off. It wasn't too bad. I made sure there was no excess liquid on my skin or around the patch. If there was liquid, it meant all the medicine did not go in and I would have to have another one put on. Later that night I started having pain along my spine. It was so bad I could not walk. We didn't know what to do so we called the on-call number. The office returned my call immediately. I was told to take the strongest pain medication that I had on hand. She explained that chemo lowers white blood cells and the injection that was given was trying to replenish those cells, so they were being pulled from everywhere. The injection causes joint or bone pain. Thankfully I had a prescription pain medication from the surgery. That was some serious pain! She told me to buy some Claritin for allergies and to take them for the next couple of days. She advised me to also take Claritin a couple of days before my treatments to help with the pain. It really did help because I did not have pain like that with my other treatments. I also had nausea along with the pain, so I took the nausea medicine prescribed and it helped right away. Mark brought me cool towels to put on my neck and head. He was such a trooper trying to do everything he could to make me comfortable. We were both scared, but the pill kicked in and the pain subsided. We were able to return the phone call to our friends who had called to check on us. They gave us encouraging words and prayed with us. So over the course of the next week, I had diarrhea most days. My temperature spiked a couple of times. Nausea kicked in a couple of days. I was able to eat lite foods and I drank plenty of liquids. There were some rough days though where anything I ate or drank came back like water. I was still hungry though. I was thankful that I still had an appetite. I was told I may lose my sense of taste or smell or just not want to eat. At the hospital, I was told that when using utensils, I may taste the metal so to be prepared to use plasticware to eat.

Having nausea and diarrhea continued for the next couple of weeks. It happened all at different times. I made sure I did what I could to stay hydrated. I was learning the smell of certain things could bring on nausea. I could eat the food and it would stay down but the smell of it nearly did me in. Sometimes I would need to hold my nose so that I could get it down. I would try to drink Ensure, but I needed to have it cold, almost frozen like a slushy so that I could tolerate the smell, and even then, I would use a straw. It was trial and error when it came to food and drink. It got costly but we did what we had to do. Each hurdle I overcame, I gave thanks to God because he saw me through it. During the next three weeks, each day was different. I had a virtual appointment with the doctor to see how things were going since treatment. I told the doctor I had some mouth soreness and diarrhea. He stated that some people develop mouth sores and that mouthwash could be prescribed. He ordered medication for diarrhea. At this time the world was being shut down because of the coronavirus. After my 1st treatment, I was debating if I would be able to attend church. I had already decided I would sit away from everyone. little did I know I would not be going to church for quite a while. I didn't know that church would not be the same from then on. The church doors, jobs, schools, stores, banks, etc. all closed. We were under a mandatory shutdown. I couldn't believe it, this was everywhere. Not only did my life change because of the cancer diagnosis and treatment, the world was also undergoing many changes. We were in a global pandemic.

Three weeks went by so fast, that it was time for treatment number two on April 2, 2020. We were on the road again, appointment time 7:30 AM. This time when we got to the hospital we were met with changes. Because of the pandemic, Mark was no longer able to go in with me. I still had to be escorted to the check-in area. Labs were drawn and I proceeded upstairs to the treatment floor. I settled in and began the waiting process for the results of my lab work. In the meantime, Mark was waiting in the parking lot to make sure I would be able to get treatment before he drove back. Since everything was shut down, he had no choice but to go back home. Once given the okay for treatment I called Mark to let him know he could go home. During each treatment, he would make 4 trips per day.

Treatment started, fluids, premeds then chemo. It made for a long day with no one to talk to. Thankfully the nurses made conversation each time they came through. I guess since my nerves were shot, I didn't sleep as much. I watched some tv, did some reading and whatever to entertain myself. Finally, it was time to call Mark so he could come back to pick me up. In the meantime, the last bag of medicine was hung. My port was flushed and the Neulasta was put on so I could get my shot the next day. The nurse reminded me of things to look for or if new symptoms developed. She again cautioned me about the use of razors on my body or getting pedicures/manicures. If possible, avoid them at all because any nick or cut could cause a lot of bleeding. I understood that loud and clear; you did have to worry about me doing any of that. Mark was waiting when I got outside. I was tired and hungry. I didn't eat much of the food they had for lunch, it wasn't appealing at the time. I was trying to cope with the changes in my body and how I was feeling. I tried eating and getting as much nutrition as possible along with plenty of liquids.

On Saturday, out of the goodness of her heart, my supervisor came over to help me with my wig as I didn't know when I might need it. She did a good job cutting the lace off of it. I appreciated her help. The days passed– some better than others. Each day I was trying to adjust to the new way of life, as it was at the time. We had never witnessed a total shutdown before nor had we ever been through a pandemic. Everybody had to stay home, there was no visiting anyone. Stores limited the number of people they could let inside at a time. People not only wore masks but also wore gloves. Everything was being sanitized. There was no public transportation available. Medical offices and hospitals were overloaded with sick people. So many people were dying! Funeral homes were at capacity and refrigerated trucks were being used to store the bodies.

My doctor advised me to limit my contact with people as much as possible because my immune system was compromised from the treatments. I coped with the side effects of treatments. Some days I felt so bad. I can't describe it. I just felt bad all over from head to toe. I kept praying and God answered each prayer. Now it is Good Friday, and I am feeling somewhat better. We had no plans, but I wanted to enjoy it as much as possible. It was after that 2nd treatment, and I wanted to try to do something with my hair. Well, I found out I couldn't even put it in a ponytail. It had been gradually coming out. Now it is by the handful. I looked at myself in the mirror and I saw bald spots here and there. I got somewhat emotional. So, I had myself a good cry and I got myself together. I called Mark into the bathroom so he could cut my hair and shave it off. He was like, "are you sure?" Yes, I was sure. I didn't know how I would look but I had accepted the fact that it had to happen. It was almost a relief when it was over because I was more stressed seeing it come out so fast. I had a wig, scarves, and a hat with hair on it. People questioned how do you feel with no hair? What are you going to do now? Me not having hair was the least of my worries. I was in the fight of my life. Sure, I missed it, but I adapted to it. It was my new look for a while.

Since we were still in the midst of a pandemic I did not see as many people, so I didn't get all the stares and questions from people. I was able to be at home and not have to worry about how I looked. Because of the risk of infection, things did not work out in my favor to be at work. Since it was apparent that I was not going to be able to go back to work as much as I wanted to, I accepted the fact and knew God would provide. No matter what I tried, I was unable to get unemployment. There was always some loophole, some criteria I did not meet…but God. God would provide in ways I did not expect. With my new look, I enjoyed the Easter weekend and celebrated the resurrection of Jesus Christ.

Time passed and it was time for my treatment #3. One of the nurses explained to me why sometimes I felt so bad around the 3rd day after treatment. It was because one of the medications given. The medication pulls from your body; trying to bring up your white blood count. It's doing its job, but it makes you feel so bad in the meantime. I was encouraged to drink plenty of water. One night after this treatment I felt so bad. I could not talk…couldn't cry or move. My husband was right in bed beside me. I couldn't alert him to let him know I wasn't well. I tried to pray or hum a song and couldn't do it. All I could do was think in my mind, "Lord have mercy on me." I kept thinking that over and over in my mind. I laid there with my mind on Jesus. It was "woman down". I can't explain it. If anyone says you are never too sick to pray, I beg to differ because I've been there. It's my truth. Early the next morning I began to feel a smidgen better. I felt my change come through. I thanked God for seeing me through even though I couldn't speak it from my mouth. God knew my heart and heard my cry. I will continue to give God the praise. When I call on God, he'll come to my rescue and yours too.

My sense of smell became heightened; everything seemed to make me nauseated. Seems like everything bothered me. I was so glad to have my nausea medicine. I kept that bottle close at hand. Can I say, never take for granted the ability to eat and enjoy your food! I was always hungry but not always able to tolerate it because of certain smells. I made up my mind– I was not giving up. I continued to trust God. By the time I was beginning to feel a little bit like myself it was about time for treatment #4. I was a little more prepared this time. Mark was getting used to taking me and leaving me there and coming back home and then later driving back to pick me up. Things were becoming familiar as far as the procedures for the day. I was thankful my lab work came back looking good, so I was ready to start treatment for the day. Mark went home. I slept some while receiving the premeds. I occupied my time by reading the bible: devotionals. Occasionally someone would text me to check on me or send something uplifting. I appreciate it all. I would sleep some more. I learned to take my own snacks because I just didn't tolerate the lunch that was served very well. It was good to hear when the nurse would come in and say this is the last bag to hang then we can get you ready to go. Of course, when I called Mark most times, he was already on the road heading back to the hospital. I'm so thankful for my husband.

Upon getting home I was tired and hungry, but grateful another treatment was behind me. Today was a day of reflection. I also celebrated my mom's birthday, oh how I wish she could be here with me. This is one time I need and want my mama. Even if it's just her holding my hand and giving me an encouraging word. She may not have been able to take this journey for me, but just having her by my side would have been enough. Seems like after each treatment I just needed to come home and get in bed just for a while. Sometimes I would go straight to sleep other times I would just lay there with my eyes closed talking to God and thanking him for bringing me through another treatment. Keeping me safe and protecting me from the virus. Even though it's been hard, I continued to trust God. It's been scary not knowing what to expect next. Not only being diagnosed with this disease, but dealing with the effects of the pandemic: No visitors, I'm not working, most businesses are closed. I wouldn't want to be out there too much anyway because this virus was taking people out so quickly. It's spreading so fast. As the weeks go by, I continue to try to stay strong and positive. God has been so good. He has put people in my life right when I need them. People who I have never met have reached out to me. The family whom I've not heard from in a long time have sent positive messages. I appreciate each and every one.

I noticed my weight was fluctuating. I guess because sometimes I can keep food down and sometimes I could not. I tried my best to stay hydrated. I was coming up on the 5th treatment. I could see the light at the end of the tunnel. As I prepared for this next treatment, I asked God for strength, for his covering and protection. Not only for me, but for Mark who has been my caretaker. I prayed for the doctors, nurses, and anyone who had a hand in my care. It had been a trying time but God. To our surprise when we went for my 5th treatment Mark was allowed to go in with me. Some of the restrictions had been lifted. I was one happy person just to have him in the room with me. I had my snacks and entertainment. Mark had to borrow some of my entertainment as he was used to not being able to be with me. It was good to have him there. I used that time to reach out to other people who I knew were going through their own storms of life. I would perhaps send a card or text just to let them know I was thinking of them. How many of you know that when you are going through something if you reach out to others to encourage them, it takes your mind off yourself for a while. It's a good thing to do for other people. I know how I feel when someone reaches out to me, and I hope I can pass that feeling along to someone else. I ask God daily to give me a word or something to someone to help them along their way– even if the word just puts a smile on their face.

With treatment #5 behind me, I was happy to know that I had only one more to go. Two days after treatment #5 I was feeling the usual effects but this time something was different. I was having shortness of breath, my legs felt very heavy when I walked, and more tired than usual. This went on Saturday and Sunday. Monday morning, I called the doctor's office. They told me to come in, they were able to get me seen for an echocardiogram and an EKG. Both tests were done on Monday. I was still not feeling my best. It was hard to even walk short distances. Later that week on Wednesday I had a virtual appointment with my doctor. He stated that since I was still having shortness of breath, he was scheduling me for a CT scan that day. He wanted to check to see if I had blood clots in my lungs. I began pleading the blood of Jesus. After my call, I texted my aunt to ask her prayer group to include me in their prayer session with my specific prayer request. I knew they would be having prayer that day. Once I arrived at the hospital, I had the CT scan completed. Afterwards I went over to the doctor's office to wait for the results. Although the walk wasn't far, I was completely tired by the time I got to the office. While waiting for the results I continued to pray and petition God for good results. The results come back showing no blood clots in my lungs. Hallelujah, praise God! The doctor suggested I go to the ER to get checked out since I still had shortness of breath and was not feeling well. I was very skeptical about going to the ER because of the pandemic and how fast the disease was spreading. I got hooked up to the IV, lab work was done, and it showed my potassium and magnesium levels were low. I was also dehydrated. I had a lot going on. I thought, wow, here I was trying so hard to drink plenty of fluids to keep that from happening. I guess in the past couple of weeks when I had diarrhea off and on played a big part in that. I was putting out more than I was putting in. I was given a potassium pill. Fluids were given, then the potassium drip was started. Let me tell you, anyone who's had potassium, by IV drip, knows how much it can burn going in. Especially when they're pushing it fast. Time went by. It was determined I would be admitted to the hospital. This was not the news I was expecting. Of course, Mark could not stay, he could not even go up to the room with me. Since I was prepared to stay, he was told he could bring me an overnight bag. That meant him going back home and coming back to Florence. Meanwhile, I was taken upstairs. I was told I would be going to the Covid floor until I could be tested and receive a negative result. That floor was so isolated and very sterile looking. All of the room doors were closed. I only saw a few staff who were dressed in full protective gear from head to toe. First thing when I got to the room, I was given the covid test. It was my first test, so I didn't know what to expect. It felt like that swab was up to my brain. Anyway, Mark brought my overnight bag to the security desk. The nurse informed me she would bring it to me. Mark made his way back home.

I was thankful to have some comforts from home: my bible, some personal items, etc. I got to thinking how blessed I was because I was not on a ventilator. I was able to do for myself. Even though I could not see out of the window or the door. I only had contact with the staff when they brought medication to me or my meals. I was glad to have my phone to be able to communicate with the outside world. I was grateful to be able to talk to family and friends. Everyone gave positive words of encouragement. I had a lot of quiet time to reflect on the past couple of months. So much had changed in and about my life. I wasn't able to sleep as much as I thought I would. My mind and thoughts were on 10. I kept praying and communing with God. Asking for guidance and direction. On Thursday evening I was told everything was looking good. My potassium level was coming up. My heart rate was much better. I wasn't dehydrated like I was upon being admitted. The covid test result should be in the next day. That would determine if I would be discharged or not. I was excited about the possibility of going home. I was very hopeful. Come Friday great news: the covid 19 test was NEGATIVE! Look at God! Everything else was still looking good. I got my discharge papers. I couldn't wait to call Mark. Mark was at the hospital before the discharge papers were completed. He did not have a problem waiting in the parking lot. Although the staff treated me well, I was happy to be going home. Happy and blessed that God brought me out. Even though I did not often see people, I had some faithful people call me regularly. One particular person would call on Friday night. I would look forward to those calls. We would talk for hours. Our spouses would go to bed on us once they realized we were talking to each other. Those calls did a lot for me.

During the week after being discharged, I was still feeling somewhat tired. It was coming up on my 6th treatment which was scheduled to be the last one. Because I was still having some shortness of breath my oncologist canceled the treatment and scheduled me to see a cardiologist. He scheduled me for an echocardiogram and a stress test. He adjusted my blood pressure medication and gave me something to help control my heart rate. Just when I thought things were going well, something else comes up. I spoke life into myself. I am going to get through this. As usual, I spoke my favorite scripture, "I will not die but live to declare the works of the Lord," (Psalm 118:17). That's one scripture I had been holding on to for the duration of my journey. Both doctors were concerned about my heart as I didn't have these symptoms or side effects before. I was praying there was no damage to my heart. Possibly chemo-related as chemo had effects on every part of the body. The oncologist termed it chemo fatigue. I continued to pray and kept trusting God. I was trying to get FMLA paperwork taken care of. Seems like there were all kinds of stumbling blocks. It was hard doing everything by phone or email. Sometimes not receiving a response at all or when I got a response I was directed to reach out to someone else because now someone else was handling it. FMLA was approved for a portion of the time. The portion of time covered was from the chemo dates, but did not include the surgery and the time after surgery.

Well, I had the echocardiogram as well as the stress test. I had never had a stress test before. I didn't know what it would entail. The cardiologist told me I would not be walking on the treadmill, but it would be done by IV because I was already dealing with shortness of breath, he did not think I could do the treadmill. The technician explained everything as she went along. Then the doctor came in and explained how I might feel. For the most part, everything went well. After the test was administered, I was told my heart rate would get higher but should eventually come down. If not, they would have to give me the reversal medication. Let me tell you, as I lay on that table, I began to feel so bad. I began to think about all sorts of things. I didn't think I was going to make it. My husband was right around the corner in the waiting area. I was thinking I was not going to be able to tell him goodbye. He didn't know what going on. I prayed to God, please don't let me die. The nurse was nearby as she said she would be. I motioned to her I needed help. She got the doctor immediately he came in and gave me the reversal meds. He told me I would feel better shortly. While lying there, I thanked God for being there with me. I was glad when that was over. When I told Mark what happened he could not believe all that was going on. It made me realize even more how fragile life is. I was so grateful to make it home. Now I had to wait on the results. Upon meeting with the cardiologist and oncologist. The oncologist determined I would not receive the 6th treatment. He felt it was too much for my body. I even had areas on my thumbnails where it appeared the blood could come right through the thin area of the nail bed. The cardiologist would not give approval for surgery until after the test results were received. I had my next scheduled appointment with a breast surgeon oncologist and the plastic surgeon. In speaking with the surgeon, she explained the procedure and what was expected to take place. She told me she would test lymph nodes, which meant they would be taken to see if the cancer had spread. I was again calling on the name of the Lord. She went on to explain the gist of the surgery. She said who all would be in there and depending on what I decided about reconstruction, the plastic surgeon would come in as well. The plastic surgeon and his assistant took measurements and pictures. So much was discussed. Scenarios were given of what could happen during the surgery that could delay reconstruction. He explained that if for some reason I lost too much blood, at the time of surgery, expanders would be put in then I would have to come back to have reconstruction done. If expanders were needed, then I would return to the office periodically to have them inflated gradually to get to the size desired. The other option would be to get implants. After a couple of days, I received the results from the stress test. Nothing was found, my heart was functioning well. Praise God, that was such good news. The cardiologist gave clearance to have the surgery date scheduled. So, then surgery was scheduled for July 29, 2020. Now I'm trying to keep myself healthy staying hydrated, managing my weight, and staying safe from getting any type of infection. I was also preparing mentally. After all this surgery for me would be life-changing. I continued to pray for peace and guidance. I was thankful for family and friends who continued to give me support and encouragement. I looked forward to the weekly family and friends' corporate prayer call every Monday night. We prayed together, worship in songs and scripture. We shared praise reports and prayer requests. Not only did the doctors want to make sure I was heart healthy they, also wanted to make sure there was enough time between my last chemo treatment and the surgery date I was thankful for feeling some better since my last treatment. I remained hopeful as the time for surgery was approaching fast. The night before my surgery, friends, and family got together on a conference call for a special prayer for me for healing and a safe surgery the next day. It was a powerful prayer of intercession. I really don't think either of us slept too much that night. We were on the road very early to Charleston. Upon arrival, I was to have a small procedure prior to surgery where the dye was inserted into my lymph nodes so during the surgery the surgeon would know which lymph nodes to take to be tested. Prior to arriving for surgery, I was given instructions on how to cleanse my body, and what medication to not take. I was told Mark would not be able to be with me prior to surgery. They would notify him when the surgery started and when I got to the recovery room. It was expected that I would stay overnight but possibly he would have to stay in the waiting room or get a hotel room. I was prepped for surgery, and met with the surgeon, anesthesiologist, and all other pertinent people who would be in the operating room with me. I was praying all the way through each step. I briefly remembered getting to the operating room and the doctor reassuring me that everything would be okay. That medication they had given me was working quickly. I don't remember counting. Praise God the surgery went well. There were no complications. Since I had decided not to have reconstruction, or have implants put in, the plastic surgeon did not have to come in. It was a blessing to hear no cancer in the lymph nodes. To God Be The Glory! That was such a relief! Although I was still feeling the effects of the anesthesia, I was alert enough to praise God. I thanked God for bringing me safely through the surgery. I woke up to see my husband sitting right there beside me in the recovery room. God is so good! I had this surgery during the middle of the pandemic when things were uncertain. The hospital was so full that I had to spend the night in the recovery room. There were no rooms available on the floor. God fixed it so that Mark was allowed to stay with me that night. I was shown how to take care of my drain tube, emptying and measuring the contents of the drain tube. I would have to do this once I got home. I also had to monitor the amount of drainage each time it was emptied, and the color of it. The nursing staff got me up later that day to walk around and to go the bathroom. So, my meal was brought to me. You know I was still feeling the effects of the anesthesia, so I started eating and fell asleep. Mark had to wake me up and tell me to chew and swallow my food. I thought I was doing that. He said he got a good laugh off of me that day. I slept well.

The next morning physical therapy came and worked with me. They gave me information to bring home to work on exercises for my arm. I was discharged and sent home with all sorts of information, and phone numbers in case of an emergency, or if I had questions after surgery. I guess I was feeling good since the medication had not worn off yet. I could tell Mark was relieved that the surgery was behind us and we were headed home. Now time for the healing process to begin. The days following surgery were not too bad. I had the expected soreness, even when the really good pain meds wore off, I wasn't in too much pain. I didn't have to take the prescription medication. Praise God for that. I had to start working on the exercises that were given to me by physical therapists. Mark was my accountability partner. He was right there with me doing the exercises with me. It was painful but I knew it must be done. I didn't want my arm to be stuck by my side from where the lymph nodes were taken. I had to get accustomed to sleeping on one side for a while. Seems like there was no comfortable sleeping position. The fluids were coming out well through the drain tube. You see this was my first major surgery, so I never had drain tubes or had to deal with them. Mark of course helped me with that as well. He took the measurements and helped to empty it as well. It was kind of in an awkward place for me to reach. The pandemic was still going on. So many people were getting infected, so many were being hospitalized and even more, were dying. We were still in shut down mode. No visitors, which I was kind of glad about. I didn't have to get dressed or put on a wig or scarf. I could just be me and take my time getting used to the new me and a new way of life for myself. I kept the drain tube for a couple of weeks before going to have it removed. The doctor explained that the hole will gradually close up on its own. My incision from the surgery was healing slowly but without complications. It amazed me that it was such a wide incision. I'm thankful that there were no stitches that would have to be taken out. The surgeon said I was healing nicely. As the weeks went by, I continued with my exercises. By doing so it would help me when it came time for radiation.

The healing process continued. I still could not lay on my left side, but I had become used to finding a comfortable position to sleep in. Sometimes it meant sitting up. I was grateful for my husband who was very patient with me. I still had days when my energy level was low. I had some days with nausea. I was limited on what I could lift. I kept praying, staying in the word as the enemy would creep in with doubt and fear. I know God does not give us the spirit of fear. I was so thankful for those people who would reach out to me by phone, text, email, or drop off a package at the door. I really appreciated their thoughtfulness. I had to do what I had to do to stay positive and also be somewhat active physically. Since the public health emergency was in full effect, the world we lived in had changed so much. We had to adapt to new ways of doing many things. Virtual doctor's appointments, virtual school, and church services were virtual. I was so thankful for my Monday night family zoom call. I looked forward to each Monday night for the prayer call. It provided hope and encouragement for whatever we were and are going through. Mark and I busied ourselves at home as much as possible. Although he was home, he still had to work during the day. I kept up with my exercises, and busied myself with reading, journaling, doing puzzles, and cleaning.

I am more than grateful for my husband. I can not put into words my gratitude for him. He took on the role of my sole caretaker. He did it all with a smile and grace. He definitely lived up to our marriage vows, in sickness, and in health. Some may say that is his obligation. That's what he's supposed to do. That may be true, but I didn't take it for granted. Many women did not have the care from their spouses as I had. So yes, I am going to sing praises to him, I am going to give him his flowers while he is living. He's going to know how much I appreciate him. This is not something I take for granted. This is not something he had to do. He's attended each of my appointments.

Even when he's not allowed to go inside. He's been a nurse, cook, maid, errand runner, and shopped for things I needed after surgery. I continued to give God thanks as each day passed. I had a couple of follow-up appointments with the surgeon. She stated that my healing was going well. I also saw the plastic surgeon one more time. Although I had decided not to do reconstruction, he still offered options. He wanted me to know that it's hard to do reconstruction after radiation. Radiated skin does not stretch well. It was thru much prayer to make the decision not to do so.

I had my initial appointment with the radiation oncologist. A whole lot of information was given. I asked a whole lot of questions. This would be different from the chemo. I was told what the steps would be leading up to the start of treatments. Eight weeks after surgery I was given the okay for radiation to begin. I went to the appointment, at that visit I got the markings on my body and x-rays and all that was needed to begin. I was also given my start day for the 30 treatments scheduled. The treatments would be daily. I was given the cream to use on my skin. I was told some things to expect once treatment got started. It was explained to me that I may have fatigue after treatments, the area may burn and get irritated as well as darken. My birthday came and I was thankful God allowed me to see it. I was celebrating life like never before. What a blessing to see my birthday. Treatments started and I adjusted to the schedule. I had not started back to work yet. I was glad I was diligent in doing my exercises with my arm. I had to be in a particular position for a certain amount of time. It was a little uncomfortable at first, but I adjusted to it. My arms got tired from time to time. As I lay on that table each day I continued to pray and give God thanks for how far he brought me. It was a new season in my life. I held onto the hope that my complete healing would come.

By the 2nd or 3rd week of treatment, I had returned to work. It felt strange being back at work after being out for 7 months. I had a new supervisor and some of my co-workers were no longer there. Before the treatment started, my hair had just started to come in a little. I was gaining a little weight too. I was thankful God allowed me to be able to have my treatment time late in the afternoon so that I would be able to go home afterward. Those days that fatigue did kick in I was glad to be able to go straight home.

So, along the way, I had been introduced to some wonderful ladies. I had only met the first few by telephone. These ladies knew all about cancer. They too had been on the journey. It was great to have someone to talk to that knew what you were going through or would have to face.

Thankfully these treatments did not cause so much sickness. My skin was beginning to darken slightly, and some of the areas were tender. I would still have occasional nausea from time to time. I was happy to be out and about a little more. I was still very cautious about being around too many people. I still limited the places where I would go. We were still not back in church, so it was so good to be able to view online service. I kept the faith and persevered. As treatments continued my skin did go through the changes where it began to burn and discolor. At least I was warned about the possibility of it happening. I took it in stride knowing that it would soon be over. Each visit probably lasted 20 minutes. The treatment itself did not hurt when being administered. All of the staff was kind and friendly and helpful with questions that I had along with suggestions as to how to take care of my skin. Along with the creams that were given, cooling patches were also given to provide relief. I'm grateful for each person who helped along the way. Time went on and I was down to my last week of treatment. THANKFUL, GRATEFUL, BLESSED. It was such a good feeling to know I was at the end of that particular part of my treatment journey. I got to ring the bell… woo-hoo! Mark and those nice ladies that I met were waiting outside with balloons, flowers, and gifts of love showing their support. It was an awesome feeling. I was ecstatic to see everyone there. I couldn't stop smiling, praising, and thanking God. As I look back over those 7 months I couldn't but help but see how my faith had grown. I realized I had to put my trust in God. When I felt like no one was there for me God said, "I am here." When I got to thinking why was I not hearing from my friends or when I would try to reach out to someone that was not available. God showed me he wanted me to totally depend on him. I got the lesson and I understand. Time went on, I had follow-up appointments with the oncologist and the radiation oncologist. I was told my skin would heal and my natural color would come back.

One of the young ladies I met referred me to a company where I could get prosthetics and custom-made breast forms and other supplies. I was still learning to adjust to this new part of my life. My clothes no longer fit the same. I had to be mindful of the style of clothing I purchased, especially tops— no plunging necklines. Choosing the right fit clothing makes a difference. I had my initial appointment with the fitter. She took some measurements and basic information was given. Nothing was ordered at the time because I needed to wait for more healing plus, I still had some swelling. When the custom breast form is ordered you want to be as close to your original size as possible. The staff at the business was so friendly and accommodating. It was a relaxing atmosphere. The person assisting me made me feel like family. I had a few more weeks to wait before everything could be ordered. I didn't realize so much was entailed in this process that would add to my level of confidence when I got dressed. It brought hope to me that I could still have some type of shape to my body. Even though a part of me was gone. If I did not tell it no one had to know at least not by looking at me. A girl still wants to look good in what she wears. With or without breasts we are still beautiful. I continued to work and tried to get back into the swing of things. Life was different now. The world was still in a pandemic. I still had to be very careful about being around others. My immune system was still compromised. The holidays were approaching, and they would be celebrated differently. Pretty much we celebrated at home. Mark and I did our thing and were grateful to just be alive and witness the day. We had so much to be thankful for. We were able to celebrate virtually with family as well. That was different, but fun. We all shared our desserts and gave thanks. Christmas came and we made the best of it; thanking God for Jesus and celebrating his birth. As the new year approached, I knew I would have to start another set of treatments. This was part of my treatment plan from the start. My initial oncologist was no longer with the practice, so I had to get used to the new doctor. He went over the plans for the treatment I would be receiving. Although it wasn't the chemo received initially but was still considered a part of the chemo regimen. As it was explained to me, I had the possibility of losing my hair again. It was hard to hear since I was just getting used to having some hair again. I may experience some sickness after treatment, but it should not be like it was previously. I would be monitored by having an echocardiogram every three months. Lab work would be done before each treatment as it was before. This treatment was one given as a preventative measure to prayerfully lower the chance of cancer from returning. I was scheduled for 14 rounds, one treatment every 21 days just as before. It seemed like a long road ahead of me. As always, I remained prayerful. I continued with my scriptures daily. I knew if God saw me thru in 2020, he would do the same thing in 2021. God did not give us the spirit of fear, so I continued to trust God.

In January 2021 I was hospitalized for a couple of days. I was dehydrated, and had low potassium and low blood sugar. My thyroid had also gone into the hypothyroid stage, and now that medication would be added to my list. I was like, here I go again. I thought I was doing good on my own with my fluid intake and keeping my electrolytes up. Thank God for giving me the mindset to get myself checked out. It could have been worse had I not paid attention to my body and the symptoms that I was having. God was right by my side even through that time I remained hopeful and grateful. I remembered to give thanks in all things. Though my faith was tested I continued to encourage myself. My dear husband stayed by my side. He made me laugh, he held my hand. Upon being released from the hospital it was time to start the treatment process. Again, we had to wait on the insurance approval of the medication. It took a little longer than we wanted it to. How ironic is it that this treatment started in the month of March as well–just like last year.

Since I was familiar with the process, I wasn't too overwhelmed with what to expect each time. I had to make arrangements with my job to take certain days off. Treatment day and a few days after. I was accustomed to looking for what I called down days. Those were the days I did not feel so well. I did not have diarrhea like I had the first year, but I did experience nausea from time to time. Thank God for medication. These treatments were scheduled from March 2021 thru December 2021. It became a part of my routine. While getting the treatment, I tried to use my time wisely and not spend it thinking about my situation. It was a time to pray for others. There were so many people worldwide who were sick, hospitalized, and families losing loved ones. Nurses, and doctors could not even go home to their loved ones for the fear of spreading the virus to their families. First responders were overworked. Many people were out of work due to their jobs closing. People were losing their homes. I just wanted to pray for all people. I continued to work and tried to be as active as possible. I was always encouraged to get physical exercise, to stay positive, and stay hydrated. Getting ample amounts of rest was important too.

During this time vaccinations were being offered for the coronavirus. Many people were torn about getting the vaccine. After much prayer and discussion with my doctor, I decided to get the vaccine. I had to be sure not to take it too close to treatment time or after treatment. Thankfully I had no issues upon taking the vaccine. I was questioned by people about getting the vaccine since it was produced so quickly, and people were unsure about its contents. Well, my response was if I can take chemo knowing what chemo can do to your body, the loss of hair, the sickness, damage that it could do to other parts of the body, etc. By trusting in God, and exercising my faith, I was going to take that vaccine. As time went on the world as we knew it was slowly getting back to some normalcy. I was still hesitant to be around large crowds and didn't venture out too much. I continued to wear my mask and practice safety precautions. Mark and I developed a stronger relationship during this journey. We did things differently. We were more intentional with our actions and expressing our feelings towards each other. During this time, I was concerned for him as far as his self-care and mental wellbeing. After all, his sole concentration was on taking care of me and my needs. Because we were in a pandemic there was not much social interaction with others. I was happy when he was able to have some time with others. I was so thankful and grateful for him to be able to be home with me during the 7 months I was out of work. It was truly a blessing that he was able to go with me to all of my appointments even though he would have to wait outside. I continued to give God thanks for him and pray for God's many blessings upon his life. It is not easy to be someone's sole caretaker. We were getting near the end of the 14 treatments. Thankfully I was not as sick with them as the previous year, but I did develop some anxiety the days just before each of the last 6 treatments. It's like I would get fearful of what they would be like. I got to thinking about what is going to happen on the day of treatment. You would think after all the treatments I had already had I would be used to going. I know I was getting closer to the last one, but it was like it was so far away. I had to dig deep within myself and pulled on my faith to make it through. I prayed and talked with God and just spoke as many positive words as I could find. My daily words through this journey: I AM HEALED, I AM HEALTHY, I AM WHOLE. I kept saying I am walking in my healing. I am walking in my victory. December 2, 2021, was the last day of those treatments. I was one happy lady. It was a beautiful day. I was smiling all over myself. When the last bag of medicine was hung, I am like thank you, Lord! All praises to him. It was a weight lifted off my shoulders to be done with those treatments I have so much to be thankful for.

Every day is a gift. Though I may hurt, have fatigue, and don't always feel well. With God, all things are possible to them that believe. As someone told me "You Better Tell God Thank You!" Throughout this time, I've held onto hope, my faith, and my belief that I would be okay. I found out you have to put your trust in God, exercise your faith, keep positive and stay away from negativity. Someone once told me "once you win it in your mind, you can do it". That statement has stuck with me. I believed I could and would win. I found hope in my faith, my devotional time & time spent with God in prayer. The support of family and friends with their encouragement.

Here are a few things I would recommend saying to yourself on a daily base that you might find helpful.

1.) I can win
2.) I am a child of God
3.) I am healed, I am healthy, I am whole.
4.) I am loved
5.) I am brave
6.) I am strong
7.) I am grateful
8.) I will not give up
9.) I will smile even through tears
10.) I can do this
11.) I have hope
12.) I am blessed
13.) I am a warrior
14.) I have the love of God

I found healing within myself when I let go and let God. Yes, I was diagnosed with the disease, breast cancer, but that is not who I am. I am more than breast cancer. I am still me! I am still the child of God who has a purpose in this life! Having a cancer diagnosis is a part of my journey. I thank God for this 2nd chance in life. I will continue to live and thrive with all of my beings. Cancer is not my name. I am a survivor. When you encounter someone who has been diagnosed with cancer please be mindful of what you say to the person. Please do not let the first thing you say is my friend or family member, or so and so had cancer but they did not make it. Let me tell you that is the last thing we want to hear. As we all know, everyone has an appointed time when we would no longer be on this earth. Do not ask, "didn't you know something was wrong?" Please do not compare one cancer patient to another. Each person is different. Their treatments are different. Don't ask why you are having so many treatments. Please remember when someone has been through rigorous cancer treatments their life is not the same. We have many side effects. Joint pain, sleeplessness, memory loss (called chemo brain), moodiness, fatigue, and physical changes. The list goes on. Sometimes we may be unsteady on our feet. There are days when we may not feel well. Our diets change. It is a lifestyle change although we try to live as normally as possible. When our treatments are done and we are able to ring the bell we still have so much to go through. We are thankful to all who encourage us daily. We are thankful that we don't look like what we've been through. When you are unsure of what to say directly to the person—just pray. Prayer changes things.

A Reason To Smile During Challenging Times
Michele Washington

My annual mammogram was usually scheduled in the month of May. For some unusual reason, the consult for my mammogram kept getting lost in the system. Finally, in September, I got my mammogram appointment. Not suspecting that anything would be different, I went to my early morning appointment. About a week later, I received a letter stating that my recent mammography examination showed a finding that requires additional imaging studies. Didn't really think much of it because a close friend of mine had gotten one of these letters before and it was nothing. I found a lump years ago and was told to reduce my caffeine which I did. I used to drink a lot of soda, which I eventually gave up. The lump went away and no further testing was needed. This time I had no lumps, bumps, or anything noticeably suspicious to make me think I had cancer. Plus, no one in my family had breast cancer. Still thinking it was nothing, I waited patiently for my next mammogram. The nurse called me frequently to follow up to ask if my mammogram had been scheduled. She would remind me to call her if I did not hear from the hospital by a certain time. I never called her to follow up; I would always wait for her call still thinking it was nothing.

Finally, in November I got my second mammogram followed by a biopsy. In 2017 on Dec 7th, I got a call from the nurse saying the Doctor wanted to see me first thing in the morning. On the 8th of December, I made what seemed like the longest 35-mile drive to my doctor at 8 am. I was his first patient of the day, which the nurse made it a point to tell me. Knowing that the Doctor wanted to see me the first thing in the morning, I knew that couldn't be good, but I was still thinking it can't be cancer. The wait wasn't long before I got called in to see the Doctor. I honestly don't remember anything he said except, "You have cancer." Cancer??? No way! Not me! I felt numb. I could feel the sorrow in his voice. The last thing I remember is him telling me what city to get treatment. I don't remember much more about the visit. My brain was trying to process my cancer diagnosis.

Who should I call first? Before leaving the building, I made the call to someone I knew would be uplifting. I did not need someone who was going to be sad with me or feel sorry for me. During the call, I realized I now had many questions? For example, what stage is my cancer? What are my treatment options? Then I had to figure out who else was I going to tell, how, and when. I chose to tell the majority of the people after I found out my treatment plan or, in other words, after the holidays. This was one of the times I wished I could have my father to talk to.

Because my diagnosis happened so close to Christmas and New Year, I decided it was best to tell the rest of my family and friends after the holidays. My first appointment with the surgeon was in January. I decided to share my news with some family and friends afterward. At my appointment, I found out I had ductal carcinoma and I was ER-positive, stage 0. I didn't know breast cancer came in so many types. Because of the location of the cancer, there was a question about the type of treatment. It was ultimately decided that radiation would be the best treatment.

Treatment began with a lumpectomy on the last day in January. I am thankful for those who were there with me on the day of my surgery. I had people drive from other states just to be there for me. Radiation was supposed to take place no later than six weeks after surgery. Four months later is when radiation would eventually take place after numerous nasty and threatening phone calls from the clinic. I went to every appointment I was scheduled for but kept getting phone calls saying I didn't. I finally told one young lady to put in my records that I don't know what she was talking about because I went to every appointment that I was scheduled to go to. I was thankful for this young lady because she got to the bottom of the situation. She got my Doctor on the phone who admitted he got distracted and forgot to put my consult in for my radiation treatments.

Everything happens for a reason. My treatment being delayed turned out to be a blessing. I happened to tell a friend who had just relocated back to South Carolina about my treatments. I thought I could handle driving myself to and fro. My drive was 45-60 minutes one way, depending on traffic. The end of the first week was brutal. The radiation Doctor did warn me about fatigue, but I didn't think it would be that bad. He said it would last about a month. Wrong! The fatigue lasted over 4 months! Naps were often part of my daily routine about 1 o'clock every afternoon for months for a couple of hours.

After my 2 hour naps, I would restart my day. I had friends who would try to discourage me. I had to remind them that the Doctor told me I had to live life as close to normal as possible. For example, I was told to continue to do volunteer work and exercise. I just needed to know my limits. Therefore, I continued, barely slowing down. I didn't realize how taxing 20 radiation treatments could be on a body, but hardly anyone knew what I was going through or how exhausted I was.

Life during and after cancer treatment wasn't easy for me, but I am grateful for those who made it easier for me to get through. I chose not to tell many people until years later. I just did not want anyone to feel sorry for me. The people who knew about my diagnosis willingly stepped up to the plate without me asking. For example, people willingly gave up their time by making meals, praying, calling to check up on me, or giving me rides in the middle of the day when I was fatigued, just to name a few things that I will forever be thankful for. Also, the day I got my radiation treatment plan was also the day I found out I was going to be a grandmother for the 3rd time, which was definitely encouraging. This gave me a reason to smile during a challenging time.

I Understood My Assignment
Chelia Frank

My name is Chelia and most people don't pronounce it correctly so I go by Lia to avoid the chopped and screwed pronunciation some people do. Growing up in Irvington, New Jersey gave this 80s baby that spunk and street smarts along with the nickname shortly Chelia. I'm still kinda shy, but I was always able to get my point across. Upon moving to South Carolina, I quickly learned a different type of appreciation for southern hospitality. At times I could be a woman of a few words and do what I call just going with the flow kinda vibe. And when the moment arises, the northern flare will ignite a flame called Lee Lee.

Being the baby of four older siblings, two being DJs, the love for music is second nature to me. It's nothing like some good early weekend morning jams while cleaning or riding down the highway. I'm always asking my kids to show my non-dancing self some new dance moves, and they of course laugh every time. Having what I call a Harley man has given me a love for loud bikes and cruising, so in his spare time he will crank up his street glide and I am not trying to get left so I have begun to learn to ride especially after he brought me a softail. Of course, like many women shopping is a part of my therapy no matter where I am I can shop. You can often find me at my, what I call buy everything store, Walmart, at least 3 times a week. Having children, especially girls, there's always something we need. Between working, being a wife, and mother, and running a successful family business. My plate is full.

Many may struggle with their purpose in life and often question the road they are traveling. But one thing I discovered about life is you may never understand what comes next, not even according to google. Today you're living your best life and tomorrow you're hit with the news that changes everything you know. As for me, at 37 years old, this forever young, lovely brown-skinned, and educated woman enjoying life, it all began to come to halt around February 2021 when I noticed my right breast was swollen. Now at first, I thought to myself, I haven't breastfed in almost 4 years, so it's not swollen from a clogged duct. Then I thought, well maybe I'm pregnant. But that wasn't the case. So time went by and still no changes. I finally made an appointment in March to see my family doctor. I left work early that day and nonchalantly walked in for my appointment with the nurse practitioner. As she examined me, she thought it may be something to do with my hormones, but nothing major. She said to play it safe, let's just get an ultrasound scheduled. In a little less than three days, I was laying on a table talking to the tech getting an ultrasound, shortly following she asked if my doctor ordered a mammogram. I said no, and the tech then left the room to get an authorization for me to have one that day as well. Now I had always heard mammograms were not for the weak. Well, let's just say in my opinion every word of that was true. I couldn't wait for that to be over, to only find out that two days later I had an appointment for a biopsy. During my mammogram, they found a mass in my lymph nodes and breast. By the time of this appointment, I was over the techs asking the repetitive question, "are you doing ok?" As much as I wanted to reply," let's be honest, NO." Instead, I just said yes. The room was very cold and I wrapped myself as much as I could in the blanket I was given. I looked around at this machine with a monitor and saw my name at the top corner as the low lighting made the screen glow. They numbed my breast and underarm area, but with every loud click from the device to gather the tissue I could feel it. I jumped in fear from the sound. The procedure lasted about an hour, but not knowing a lot about this type of procedure, along with listening to the tech who may not have ever had this type of procedure, let alone dealing with the questions going on in my mind while trying to act normal, I went to work after my biopsy procedure and really wished I was home in my bed. My breast was very sore and I was told to rotate ice packs every hour to keep the swelling down and take Tylenol for pain. No one was fully aware of what was going on at this point besides my fiancé and a few of my coworkers. I just didn't want anyone to really worry. Until I knew what was going on. At this point, cancer was the furthest thing from my mind. I was thinking it may be a cyst and it would be an easy fix. The results would take about a week or less to come back. So the waiting game began. My parents and I normally talk every day and keeping this a secret was not easy at all. Especially when Mother's Day came. We all went out to dinner and took pictures; just having a great time. I felt like I was carrying a ton of bricks holding this secret in. I just knew at some point my mom would ask if something was going on. It was hard, but I didn't want to worry my family, especially my dad who is a prostate cancer survivor. That day the weather was perfect. We took tons of pictures to top the day off.

During a normal work day, at Sumter Pediatrics, I'm answering the phone, making appointments, and checking patients in and out. On May 25th, I was sitting at my desk when my phone lit up from a call. I stepped away from my desk to answer the call and spoke to the nurse in regards to my next appointment to discuss my results. At this point, I knew something wasn't right because she would have told me over the phone. I quickly logged onto the patient portal to see if the results were loaded up, but no luck. With the weight of this secret getting heavier, I decided during my lunch break to call and break the news to my parents, and right away my mom and dad said they

96

were coming with me for that appointment. My mother questioned me for not telling her sooner. I explained how I didn't want them to worry. On May 27th, 2021, I sat in a chair with my mom next to me waiting for the doctor to come in. What was unusual for me was instead of going into an examination room to talk to the nurse, they took us into his office. I remember looking around and saying to myself I don't think this is good but nah, it's just my mind overthinking. Then Dr. Moses, at Prisma Health Tuomey Day Surgery, walked in and sat down at his desk. It was all decorated with family pictures. He said, "Ms. Frank, it's just what I had a feeling it would be. It's breast cancer." At that moment, it felt like time had stopped. I was then diagnosed with Stage 2 invasive ductal carcinoma. Like what is this, and how, is all I could think of. At the moment, I honestly didn't hear it. I just kind of went with the conversation and shook my head as if I understood. He talked about a treatment plan and explained how this was very much curable with it being caught so early. My mom was speechless and her eyes filled with water as she looked at me. I looked away. I was trying my best not to make eye contact. I said, "ok, what do we do next?" He then explained I would need chemo, surgery, and then radiation. He also said he was referring me to a local oncologist. He handed me a book and his personal cell phone number and asked that I not google anything but just call or text him and he will answer any questions I may have. He then smiled at me and said we will get through this Ms. Frank. I smiled back and said ok and we walked out into the waiting area. I then had to tell my dad, who was in the waiting room. I told him the news in the most positive way possible, but I knew it crushed him even more to hear this. We rode the elevator in silence. I remember looking at my dad just shaking his head. But it was that day that he grew a different type of bond besides father and daughter. We would share a cancer-surviving bond. We walked to our cars. As I got in my car and pulled out, I started to feel numb. And the word death began to play in my head, but I held it together because I knew my next challenge was telling my children and fiancé. Prior to this, we were dealing with my fiancé's medical condition that had appeared suddenly a few months prior. We had just begun to get that under control. **NOW THIS!** I called him and he was working, driving his truck at the time. I said, "it's cancer". And he replied with silence. I said, "Hello?" He said, "I'm here." I asked him if he heard me and he said, "are they sure?" I said, "yes." Going back to that day and asking him why he didn't say much, he said I just couldn't process it at that moment and I didn't know what exactly to say. Things began to seem as if the blue clear sky had gotten gray and dark like a storm was approaching. Once I got home, I contemplated how to break it to my then 14-year-old daughter. At this age, knowing she was knowledgeable about this type of cancer after losing family members to it. My mom had gone to pick up my 3-year-old, Taylor, from daycare. We waited until Toni got home so I could break the news.

Once she got home I sat in the living room with her and explained my diagnosis. I tried my best to reassure her that mommy was going to be ok. And it was nothing to worry about. She said ok and seemed to be going with the flow. She played with her sister as usual. I then decided to call my manager and gave her the news while sitting in my bathroom downstairs. I started explaining and began balling my eyes out at the same time. All she could say was we will get through this. That night as I went into my bathroom to get ready for bed. My mind was all over the place, wondering what chemo would be like, how would it make me feel, or if I would survive. I then got my phone and let my worship playlist play as I prepared for my shower. As the water began to fall, so did my tears. I cried my eyes out once again. I just asked God, why me? How can I do this Lord? Please don't take me from my children! I'm begging you! Please, God! I cried in silence because I didn't want to worry my children. I grew angry and needed God to know that this couldn't be happening to me. He had to make it better. The hot water had begun to get cold and it felt like small rocks were beating on my skin. As I dried off and came out of the bathroom, my daughter's bedroom door was open and I looked at her window. I noticed the sun was setting and the darkness of the night drew near for everyone else. The day was ending, but not for me. It had only just begun. That next morning, I was then scheduled for more tests, so back to Tuomey I went. And of course, my mom was right by my side, even though she couldn't go in the back she wanted me to know that she was right there.

Now, while waiting for one of the three procedures I was getting done that day, I sat in a waiting room that had some dim lights and hospital staff walking past every few minutes. The first lady came in, we greeted each other and she sat down. Then shortly after, two other ladies walked in. One, in particular, was wearing a breast cancer mask. I can't say how the conversation began, but we all got to talking and two of them were survivors and the other was a thriver. But it was something about this one lady that when she began talking it was like she understood! She said you will get through this, you just have to trust in God. It was as if she felt my fears and could see right through me. She hugged me. I could not do anything but cry from the relief. She encouraged me to stay strong. We exchanged numbers that day and I walked out of that waiting area feeling stronger. But the fear of the unknown was still scary. Once I got home, I grabbed my phone and began to send out a few text messages about my diagnosis. After that, my phone rang with back-to-back calls from friends and family giving me love and support. It wasn't a person I talked to and gave the news to that didn't have a silent moment on the phone. I said to everyone, "Hey I'm going to be ok! I'm going to beat this! It will not beat me!" At those times I had to realize that my positive energy was what helped my friends and family push through. Your sickness feeds off of negative energy. Later that evening, the lady I had met at the hospital sent me a text just checking on me and asked me to call her tomorrow so we could talk more. Well, from that day, my phone never seemed to stop ringing or receiving text alerts. Many times I would put my phone on silent, so I could concentrate or get rest. Now the 773 number was calling. I took a deep breath and answered. It was the nurse calling to set up my day surgery to have my port put in place. So, as Dr. Moses explained, it was going to be a pretty simple surgery.

On the morning of the surgery, as Will and I got off the elevator, I began to have a feeling that I hadn't at the time been familiar with. I was scared. This was not my first time having surgery but this one felt different. It was as if everything was happening so fast and no one was really explaining why these things were happening. The lady called my name to go back but at that time Will wasn't allowed in the back until the nurse had me prepped. Now I'm alone. I had my phone so I'm ok at this point. Then that all changed when the nurse could not start my IV. I have never been a person to be in pain from a needle, but today I felt it every time she tried and failed, the feeling that I had when I got to the hospital had now gone from a 10 to 10000. After the third try, I was literally in tears and was ready to just say forget that I'm going home and not having surgery. She then called in another nurse who was a little older. She came to the side of the bed and grabbed my hand and began to rub it and say "it's ok, we're going to get it", as she passed me a tissue to wipe my face. I laid my head back on my pillow and took a few deep breaths. My anxiety was still there, but it had begun to lower as she talked and asked me questions to take my attention away from what she was doing. As promised, she got my IV going on the first try. I didn't feel anything. As she taped and secured my IV, she said "see, I told you!" and she smiled! And then finally Will came in and sat with me while we waited for them to wheel into the operating room. That was on a Monday. I had previously had my first appointment to discuss my chemotherapy treatments the week prior, so it would be 25 rounds of chemo, once a week.

On Wednesday morning, my mom and I got the kids off to school and daycare. We then stopped to grab breakfast. Then we pulled into Santee Oncology's parking lot for my first treatment. Now I know cancer has no age discrimination, but I had to say I felt so out of place there. The first nurse called me to draw my blood, then I waited for another escort for my mom. I took my seat in their big recliner and my mom sat next to me. I looked around like, where are the TVs? My nurse, who was very nice and professional, talked about everything that I was receiving that day. And it started with some regular IV fluids and then what is called the "Red Devil'. So she then came over with something I was not prepared for. I was told they usually numb your port area, so the needle doesn't hurt much. To my surprise, the nurse informed me they did not do that there and she then pulled out a needle (one that looked huge) to access my port. I thought for sure I was on the moon when I saw stars from the pain I felt when she stuck the needle into my port. My mom was so upset with the nurse. All I could do was just look straight ahead and gasp in shock. The pain eased up as my infusion began. I reached into my snack bag and began to play crossword puzzles. My mom and I chatted while the machine did its work really fast. We were there for three hours. That day when I left, I said oh no I'm not going back there I can't do it. I had an appointment with Dr. Moses the following week and expressed my fears and why I did not want to return. He then referred me to Dr. Collins at SC Oncology in Columbia. They promptly called and set my first appointment. Unlike the others, you first had to take a class on chemotherapy. My sister Net accompanied me to my first appointment and class. Following the class, we met Dr. Collins who was very straightforward and empathic and at the same time, which I very much appreciated. He laid out the treatment plan for chemo one day and the following day I would come back for fluids. He wanted to begin right away because he did not like going too many days without treatment. Later that week, I showed up ready for my second treatment, only this time I was prepared with numbing cream for my port area. When I checked in, I was then told to head downstairs to check in that area to have my blood work and vitals done. Then the nurse escorted you to your area for treatment. I sat in a recliner and pulled the side table up. My sister pulled up a chair beside me with her bag of snacks ready for the day. My nurse came over and greeted me. She then introduced herself along with the other two nurses that would be handling my care. I was put on the front row since it was my first time there, so I could be monitored in case of an allergic reaction. Then she came with the needle, but instead of some spray to numb the area as she wiped the area clean, she says "I'm going to put a freeze spray on this area if that's ok with you?" And I said, "oh I put some cream on it before I left home because I thought y'all didn't have that". She smiled and said, "oh we know this is painful, so we try to make you as comfortable as possible." Then it was time for IV fluids and pre-meds, which included the lovely Benadryl. I got up to use the restroom and grabbed a cup of ice in preparation for the red devil.

The big difference in treatment centers was how I received the RED DEVIL. This time the nurse had it in a big syringe and slowly fed it into my IV. The whole treatment process lasted about four hours that day. I left feeling ok. My sister and I headed back to Sumter, chatting away. By the end of the week, as I stood in my bathroom mirror, I rubbed my hand across my head and wiped it clean. All of my hair was completely gone—even my eyebrows. Losing my eyebrows hurt worse than any of my hair. By losing those, it really made me look like a cancer patient, but I was determined to keep them drawn on every day. I repeated treatments every week. Between my dad and sister, they rotated taking me to my treatments. And every morning on the way there, my brother Gerald would call and give me my morning inspiration and encouragement. Then it would be followed by a text from a sister/friend asking for my location and making sure I was on track with time. By the 3rd treatment, I could feel my body wearing down more and more. The day after treatment I could barely get out of bed. Every inch of my body ached. It felt like all the wind was knocked out of my body when I tried to just take a shower on my own. My mom stayed at my house Monday through Thursday while Will worked during the week. My appetite started to change, and oftentimes I forced myself to eat. When I ate anything with grease or anything fried, it caused me to vomit. I changed a lot of my diet and cut pork and beef out and drank water the majority of the time. The treatments grew harder and harder for me each week. Each time I cried the night before. The thought of having my body go through this over and over was hard to bear. At first, I missed family functions because I didn't want to compromise my immune system and risk catching covid or any type of sickness, so I stayed in the house a lot. Plus, I didn't want to deal with the questions of how things were going with treatment or was I sure I should be eating or drinking that. Then I began to feel like my kids are missing so much so on the weekends when I felt good I wanted to just go anywhere. It didn't matter as long as they could get out of the house. More and more of my close family and friends came to visit and hang out with us. That helped a lot. Having cancer began to play a huge part in my mental stability as well as dealing with tingling and neuropathy in my hands and feet. I tried a few remedies like oils and using cold mittens on my hands and feet during treatments; tricks that I learned from a few "breasties".

As time went by, and I went to treatments and doctor appointments back to back, my body changed a lot. My skin got darker and dry. My taste buds weren't the same. And my energy was limited. After joining the ladies of Faith Strong, we formed a sisterhood that then allowed me to be able to vent and learn more about the different things that were happening to my body. On a usual, weekly doctor visit morning, I awoke feeling horrible. I was weaker than normal after treatment and couldn't keep anything down. On the drive to Columbia, I tried to eat some breakfast, but I couldn't eat a lot. Once I arrived they drew my blood as usual and the nurse took my vitals. He said,

"Hey lady, today isn't a great day." I replied with a head shake and he said, "I understand, so let's get you right". Once Dr. Collins examined me, he told me I was getting dehydrated and needed to have fluids. My mom and I headed downstairs to the infusion room. I got hooked up and started my fluids shortly after I began to vomit and feel light-headed. The nurse came and called the doctor. He ordered medicine, which put me straight to sleep. I woke an hour or two later feeling much better and we went home. My dad drives me to all of my appointments and treatments in Columbia and my mom goes to all of my appointments with my doctors, so she can be able to help me remember what the doctor says.

As time has progressed, I noticed some of my memories have changed from simple names or events. I can't remember them as well as I normally would. I learned it's called chemo brain, which is common in most cancer patients receiving chemo. After a follow-up visit, the neuropathy had gotten worse and due to the level of neuropathy I was experiencing, my oncologist stopped my treatments. He didn't want to cause further damage that could be irreversible, so with only four left, chemotherapy was over. In October, we held a ride for a cure in Sumter. I rode on the back of Will's bike. The weather was just right and it was just one of the best feelings, cruising around. Shortly after the ride, my family friends and I rushed back to my house to set up a birthday surprise Patriots theme party for Will. Everything turned out great! He was so surprised because he had no clue, let alone that I planned it in less than two weeks. Unlike other patients who get to ring the bell after their last treatment, I was unable to. So I planned for my family to do my bell-ringing ceremony via zoom. That Sunday afterward we traveled to my treatment center and I rang the bell outside. I wanted to cry, but I held back my tears in my speech on May 27th at 1:00 pm. I gave the doctors back the news they had given me. I knew God healed me and cancer picked the wrong one. I celebrated that weekend as I got ready for the next phase. I got myself prepared for a major surgery. Every Sunday my uncle Charlie and aunt Loretta would stop by for a quick second or call to pray with me. This helped me get through my toughest week when I felt like the pain was just unbearable. I would revert back to the scriptures my uncle and many others shared with me. Through everything, I never lost my faith. I knew God had his hands on me. On November 4, 2021, in the early morning hours, we walked into Tuomey. After my IV was started, I was wheeled to another floor to have another mammogram done. There were two other ladies ahead of me, so at one point I was laying in the bed in the hallway facing a lady who I was laughing with as I watched her clean out her desk. Then along with having this IV dripping, I had to use the restroom, which felt like a million times. Finally, it was my turn to go in. Next, I was wheeled back downstairs, but to a different room where I now got this painful dye injected into different spots on my breast. It was quick but painful. Shortly after I needed a different type of numbing done. Afterward, I didn't remember a thing. Dr. Moses performed my lymph ectopy and double mastectomy and Dr. Clark performed my reconstruction at the same time. I woke up in my room feeling ok. I remember looking down at my chest and saying how big my breast is now. Then I leaned forward and saw the drain tubes. No one prepared me for that part. They pulled and tugged at my sides when I moved around. Things became real for me quickly after those drains. I slept in the recliner. It was the only way I could get comfortable. The worst part was not being able to shower for almost a month because my drains could not get wet and my doctor did not want to risk me catching an infection. So I was on antibiotics the entire time as well, along with weekly visits to Dr. Clark's office that my mom had to drive me to. My non-affected breast took the longest to heal and have the drains removed. It stayed swollen and it got to a point my doctor tried to drain fluid off with a needle in her office but it did not help. A home health nurse came to see me twice a week to make sure my drains were ok and draining properly. It seemed like it took forever to finally have my drain tubes removed, but what a relief it was when they did, and to take a shower felt like heaven. Just a few weeks after that I met with yet another doctor to get a treatment plan for radiation. I was always told radiation was the easier part of things and it was going every morning, Monday thru Friday. I would come in and go into a changing room, take my top off and put on a gown, then tech comes and we go into a room that is freezing cold with a huge machine. You lay on the table and began to have your body lined up with markers that the radiologist put on me the week prior. Once you receive those they put some waterproof tape on top of them and they prefer for you not to scrub very hard in those areas. At this point, I'm saying ok, this may not be too bad. And I called Sumter pediatrics and asked to be put on the schedule a few days a week. After you get into the right position, they do a few x-rays to confirm the lasers will hit the target area exactly. It can't be off-target in any way. As the radiation begins, this huge machine goes around you and makes a hmm and clucking noise. You aren't there long enough to take a nap, so many times I would just relax and think about the day I faced ahead of me. After treatments, I went to work 3 days a week. And after I got off, I would be wiped out. I had just enough energy to pick up Taylor from daycare, fix dinner and take a shower. My bedtime was promptly between 9 and 9:30 pm. Doing this each week, despite the tiredness gave me a sense of normalcy. As radiation got closer to the end, I began to see the change in my skin. It had gotten darker and I began to get tender to touch. I was told to use a cream and Aquaphor to help with the discomfort. With only two treatments left the

103

skin on my arm and breast were raw and pink in color. I couldn't wear a bra, so I wore a tank top. By the end my skin looked horrible and hurt so bad I went to my doctor and had to get some cream for my burn. It worked wonders. I was so proud of myself for completing another milestone and getting closer to the finish line. During my visit with my oncologist, he recommended I have a hysterectomy and set me up with an appointment with my OBGYN in Sumter. I did my consultation, and shortly after I had a date for surgery. Even though I was only asked to do a partial hysterectomy I opted to do a full hysterectomy. The choice was pretty easy to make. It was either come in once a month for a year to get a hormone blocking shot along with taking a pill by mouth every day for 10 years. Or have a hysterectomy and take a pill every day for 10 years and not risk getting pregnant again and producing more estrogen and causing my cancer to come back.

On March 19th I pulled off yet another surprise, but this time for my mom's birthday we all gathered at Logan's and when she walked in and saw everyone she was shocked that I "got over on her." Because she always says she doesn't want a party and this year not to worry me. She was just happy to be alive. That Monday, March 21st, I walked into Tuomey hospital once again only this time my anxiety wasn't as bad and I prepared myself more. Everything started out good. My IV was started, and Will and I were sitting waiting for me to go back. It wasn't long before I was being wheeled down the halls when I woke up. I was in my room. The first thing I said was, "lord I made it thank you". I called my mom and was picking the kids up from school and was on the way to the hospital to see me. Toni came up to my room first. She enjoyed the free gloves and laughs we had while I Facetimed Taylor, who was in the car with my mom in the hospital parking lot. Often I would say oh my gosh I need a vacation from my kids, yet I still missed them. Toni left and shortly after Will came I fell asleep on him, he woke me saying, "I'm getting ready to head back to the house". Right after he left, the OBGYN came in and gave me some shocking news. My procedure was done, laparoscopy, and he must have nicked my bladder during the procedure, so I would have to wear a catheter for a few more days until my bladder was healed. I was pretty groggy, so I didn't really understand what he had said. I just knew I was sleepy. The next morning the urologist came in and further explained what was going on so I could really understand. I went home shortly after and on the journey of having a catheter for 10 days. Just when I began to sleep in my bed again I was back in my recliner trying to get comfortable. I had to adjust my body in different positions to get rest along with being sore from the four small incisions on my stomach. I was again unable to drive for two weeks. It felt like a year of being out of work and not having a steady income. But God made a way for me and my family every time. Will worked hard and took care of all the major bills and still provided us with extra things. Sumter Peds and 803 Nutrition really stepped in for me and raised money to help with bills and anything else I needed. I could not thank them enough for everything they did from beginning to end. While out of work I concentrated on making and designing t-shirts for breast cancer and any other requests others had. Then once having time to heal from each surgery, especially once the catheter was removed, we decided to expand our business minds after doing some successful catering for family and selling delicious treats we knew it was time for another venture. We launched our businesses full blast and added a party bus: " Fantasy 9". Many times it seemed like the days were dark and of course, death crossed my mind. Just not knowing what could happen day to day, guessing what the doctor may tell me. I stayed awake many nights having a million thoughts run through my head telling myself I am strong and I will beat this. I couldn't let my girls see me down, they needed me most. I had to be here to watch them grow up. When I was given this opportunity to share my journey I didn't know where to start writing. I knew it would be emotional, just thinking of how far God had brought me. As I began, it was always the vivid detail of the day I got diagnosed that never left my mind. I was just a normal woman living in Sumter, working and raising children like anyone else. I was no stranger to the word breast cancer, after having lost a grandmother and a great aunt to breast cancer, and aunts, cousins, and a friend surviving breast cancer. But when it is you, everything changes. At first, I didn't understand why God chose me to have breast cancer. Why did he allow this hateful disease to come into my body? Watching my hair fall out and hiding it from my family, I felt so ugly on the inside at times. When I did go out, I felt like people stared at me. I knew they really were not, it was just the thought of them looking and noticing. With covid being on the rise, I was worried about catching that and not being able to recover since my immune system was so low. I was scared to even catch a cold. I kept my children pumped up on vitamins and we sanitized the house every night along with our nightly routine. I got into wearing my wigs more and mastered drawing on my eyebrows to let the outside look better than how I was actually feeling on the inside. My oncologist also understood my feelings and came to the conclusion of starting some medicine to assist with my depression. It was these little things that made me realize how much talking to someone and letting them know when you need help really means. Along with the different changes I had I gained so much weight and it seemed like none of my clothes fit. I adapted to it and just bought clothes when I could, even if it was a simple dress. If it made Chelia feel good and look good I bought it. Will was my biggest cheerleader he never looked at me any differently. If I wanted something and it in his power he made sure I had it. Toni stepped up to be best big sister to Taylor that I could have asked for. I appreciated date nights and the quality time I spent with my family. My parents are my superheroes. They spent plenty of days driving me to appointments, taking my kids back and forth, doing whatever it took. My true friends made sure they called or texted daily if they couldn't stop by, some even took time out to drive me places when needed. The outpour of love I received from my support system was unreal. It's nothing for me to go to my mailbox and have a package, card or wake up to a cash app deposit. I hear my doorbell ring and I have flowers, edible arrangements, or a front porch full of groceries. I formed so many bonds with other fellow thrivers and survivors along my journey that I was able to share my cares and concerns. It was days that I just needed to vent and having someone that understood the road I was walking down made things just that much easier to express my feelings and emotions too. From this experience, I have learned to live life and not let anything stop me.

Yes, you may get scared sometimes and feel like you just don't understand what life is throwing at you. But trust me; God assigns us all a mission to complete. No directions just lead by his word and blind faith. There were many times it got rough. Instead of throwing in the towel I just dug deeper and fought harder. I prayed more and leaned on the word of God. The moments I felt like giving up I talked to God and he reassured me every time that he was right there with me. I put on my shield of armor and faced my battles head on. I fought for all those who lost their strength to fight who let the depression of dealing with the ups and downs and changes of cancer and what it does to your mind and body. I fought for all those that gave up because they didn't think they had enough strength to fight and their faith got weak. I fought for those who weren't able to fight and their battle was cut short. Trust in the Lord with all thine heart and lean not unto your own understanding. In all thy ways acknowledge him, and he shall direct thy paths-Proverbs 3:5-6. Along with my dad we have done cancer walks together. And these experiences as cancer survivors have strengthened our bond tremendously. We are both cancer survivors. Glory to God. The day I went to my appointment and my mom asked my doctor if I was cancer free and the doctor replied yes she is in remission. Those were the sweetest words I could ever hear. We left Columbia smiling feeling like the heaviest load had been removed and I beat it and it did not beat me! Cancer is a diagnosis no one ever wants to hear, but unfortunately, we do. I survived and vow to always educate women on breast cancer and the importance of listening to your body. And not to assume it's nothing. The more time you put it off, the worse it could be. The earlier the detection, the better. Learning many unknown cancer preventive measures is my biggest target for education and knowing what you put into your body and the long term effects it may have. From the foods we eat to the products we use everyday that contain chemicals which aid in the organisms that form into breast cancer cells. I will continue to fight, advocate, and educate every day because I am #CheliaStrong #Faithstrong #Survivor

Overdue Adoration
MaryAnn Williams

So often, we find ourselves looking at ourselves through the mirror of other people. Am I attractive? Am I fat? Am I smart? Am I good enough? The answers we give ourselves are often a validation of the opinion ingrained in us by others. A cancer diagnosis will make you take a long look at yourself. You start to answer questions about yourself from your own introspection. Looking back over my life, I see a smart, petite girl with big dreams; dreams so big they could not be defined. I grew up in a small town with a BIG family. I am the second oldest of seven. You see, we were trend-setting back then. I have a biological sister and five cousins who are my brothers. I am not sure what the modern-day term is, but we are certainly blended.

I left my small town to move to Washington, D.C. It was my mecca. I worked in fortune 500 companies and met/shook hands with some very influential folks. Yes, D.C. has been good to me. I am highly educated and earned graduate degrees. I work at the pulse of the United States government. Yes, you guessed it, I work on Capitol Hill. On any given day you could find me moving and shaking around the beltway. My hair was always on point, and my outfits were more than stylish. I did not need anybody's validation to tell me I was IT. I got dressed every day wearing confidence. I was living my life and living it abundantly.

I had begun to start maturing, some call it aging. I can remember looking in the mirror and seeing fine lines of my youth slipping away. I had begun to experience my own summers but was not too worried because I still looked good. I started feeling an uncontrollable itch in my left breast, so much so that I had scraped the skin each day trying to calm it down. Several times, in particular, I can recall moments of embarrassment. One was in a meeting where I had to excuse myself and go to the women's room to try to contain the itch. The other happened when I had planned an evening out with friends. It was summer and very hot. I came home from work to shower and freshen up. What happened next scared me to death.

While drying my body, blood began to spew out of my breast uncontrollably. Wait what is going on? Yes, it was bright red blood all over my white-tiled bathroom. I did not panic but thought ok this must have come from all that scratching. Here is where the embarrassment came; I met up with my friends only to have my blouse full of blood at the part where my nipple would be. I did not notice, or I would have changed clothes immediately. A friend brought it to my attention. The blood never skewed out anymore upon bathing, but I just recently discarded the bra where the inside of the cup went from a faint color to the covering the entire bra.

In 2017, I was diagnosed with a rare form of cancer, mucinous Stage2. After receiving this devastating news, all I could do was cry. Depression was real for me. I could not look past the diagnosis. I was paralyzed. How could it be that cancer had taken hold of my body? Days turned into weeks, and I looked up, I had wasted an entire month. Get a hold of yourself girl you have things to do, I said to myself.

I began what seemed to be an endless amount of doctors' appointments. You name it I had it done. I cannot remember where I am supposed to be or what type of doctor I needed to see. After several biopsies and expert opinions, I needed to have a mastectomy. Looks like we can treat this with just surgery and pills. Okay, I must be lucky. Or so I thought. Let us get this done doc I am ready. Oh no, Cancer said it will not be that easy. From January 2018 through June 2018, I had six surgeries. I thought that I had outsmarted cancer and said I will do a double mastectomy, never to be bothered with this again. You see this was my only child's senior year of high school. I could not have him worry about my existence and his future. It is too much for a teenager. Heck, it is too much for me. My son is so special to me, not because he is mine but because he is God's living promise of Psalm 37:4: "Delight yourself in me and I will give you the desires of your heart." I had already beaten the diagnosis of infertility through this scripture.

I walked in fearful faith. What is that you ask? It is walking fearing the worst but claiming you had faith in God's power. I was angry with God and frustrated with myself. I wish I had taken better care of my body when I was younger, watched my weight, and watched what I ate. I was angry that I was trying to do good and God had let this bad thing happen to me. Why me, Why now.

I continued to walk in the way for a while longer. I began to examine my relationships with others. I mean all relationships, friendships, "romanceships", "situationships". I had to see clearly, what I was holding on to. I wanted this life but it did not want me.

I have many acquaintances that I used to refer to as friends. This diagnosis let me know exactly who those people were. My friends, the ones that cried with and for me, offered suggestions on how together we would fight, and many hours of laughter. Those were the ones that are my friends, others said sorry to hear that, I will pray for you. This statement did not take them out of the friend category, but it opened my eyes to the mirror of how they reflected on relationships and associations.

Romantic relationships began with difficulty. When was the right time to disclose, if ever? What would be their reaction? How do you deal with the rejection? Breast cancer had robbed me of my womanhood. I did not feel complete anymore. My reconstruction surgery was not so good. My breasts were larger than what I wanted and they were just there like icing on a cake. They looked good but served no real function anymore. Body dysphoria had begun to rear its ugly head. I did everything I was advised by the doctors to do and this is what I am left with. Yuck, Yuck, Yuck.

In 2019 I felt a small lump, same breast, same spot. My thoughts, here we go again. I was hopeful that it was scar tissue. More biopsies later, I learned cancer had returned. Let us start this dance all over. This time around a shorter surgery, but radiation will be done. I underwent 32 rounds of radiation. It was a tremendous inconvenience to my schedule but not so bad. Heck, it was the beginning of the pandemic and the world was still. Time to really focus on what mattered. But yet again, I was asking myself what that might be.

I started again, looking in the mirror of other people to find my reflection. Hold up, wait a minute, this is your life woman. Yours, not others. You are kind, loving, and giving. You do not need someone else's projection to show you that. You are compassionate and smart. You are funny and fun-loving. Hey wait a minute, this is me, all of me; no validation from others needed. Girl, you finally took off your mask. All right now. Mirror, mirror on the wall, what do you see? Damn, it was a trick. I see this body bruised and cut up. A shell of what it used to be. You, yeah you, go put on some clothes to cover those scars. You are not what you used to be. This body is UGLY, UGLY, and UGLY. Well, I covered up more and more. Hid behind the camisoles and sports bra even when it was time to have adult playtime. Hey dude those things are off-limits. You cannot see them, touch them, or play with them. I am all woman but from the collarbone up and below the waist. Do not think about the midsection.

December 2021 dealt the most deviating of all blows. This cancer had metastasized to the other breast. That is not supposed to happen. I had a double mastectomy. Cancer, you will not win this fight. I was told that I am in Stage 4. I panicked and cried. I mean a lot of crying. So thankful for intercessory prayers. I have found my strength. I have found myself. I do not need others to validate me. I love my body. I accept every scar. It reminds me that I am greater than what tried to destroy me.

I had to endure 28 rounds of radiation and must take monthly injections and pills to stay alive. I trust God and his healing power. He delivered me from the stronghold of cancer. The disease that was going to extinguish me brought me more clarity and keen vision.

I have a scar on my left ankle from a childhood accident. I was told that I had fallen on a broken bottle and the cut was deep. I do not remember

111

the age or the accident itself. I now view cancer that way. I have a REAL faith walk. Joel 2:25 says I will restore to you the years that the swarming locust has eaten. I am true testimony and a miracle. I am here by God's grace, his mercy, and the love of family and friends. I am reaping the harvest of a full and enjoyable life. Do I have regrets? Sure, everyone does, but those things no longer define or paralyze me.

One might ask yourself how you find out what matters. These questions work for me.

1. Does it please God?
2. Does it bring me peace?
3. Is this my reflection or someone else's projection?
4. Is it a memory or is it a moment?
5. Am I growing or staying the same?
6. Am I choosing my circumstances or are they choosing for me?

My answer to the questions helped me redefine my life. I would always quote Jer. 29:11 For I know the plans that I have for you, declares the Lord, plans to prosper you and not harm you, plans to give you hope and a future.

I can ask myself many questions, but answers that encourage movement. My best friend would always say when you are tired you make a change, but baby when you get sick and tired, you do something! I laughed when she said that, but she put it in this context. Your car breaks down, you repair it. It breaks down again, you are tired, but you repair it. It breaks yet again, you say I am sick and tired of this car breaking down, so you make a choice to either go without or get a different one. Sick you can play around with but, being sick and tired requires immediate action. There is certainly no joy in receiving this diagnosis, but I am reminded of God's word. In James 1:4, we find these powerful words, "My brethren, count it all joy when you fall into various trials, knowing that the testing of your faith produces patience. But let patience have its perfect work, that you may be perfect and complete, lacking nothing.

Today, I walk with a boldness of not only not looking like what I have been through, but also marching to my own beat. My faith is fearless and unmovable. I had an aunt who recently passed away after being on hospice for greater than three years. She was very special to me. She had a mantra that she lived by. I use it to this very day. She would say, "**Wake Up To Live**". Before cancer, I was existing. Sure, I was doing things but now b-a-b-y I am living! I am making memories and expanding my friend circle. I mentioned earlier that I had acquaintances in the past. This expansion of friends is just those friends. Nothing but positive energy. We build memories. We talk about tomorrow but we live for today. I often joke with them that death might catch me, but when it does, it will find me living.

I no longer wear a mask to fit the picture that I think others see of me. When you see me, what you see is what you get. I am not rude or braggadocious. I am happy and content. I find joy in being myself; the weight I was carrying around to please others had just got too heavy to carry and was not necessary.

I often borrow a line from two of my favorite Poets. Langston Hughes, said, "Life for me ain't been no crystal stairs". Maya Angelou, said, "I am a woman Phenomenally. Phenomenal woman, that's me."

I Answered The Call
Stacey Haywood

Oh, what a night! The blood was pumping wildly through my veins. My palms were sweating, as I waited for my name to be called. Every seat was filled; the crowd rowdy with praise. This was it. My calling was fulfilled. I was about to preach my initial sermon. I can recall thinking to myself, having answered this call three years prior, *has this moment really arrived?* As I heard my name called, and stood to mount the platform, the night became electrifying! April 12, 2000, a night of destiny, a night of change, and a night of fulfillment in my life. I preached hope, belief, and prayer; little did I know that I would be preaching to the choir that night with a sermon titled "Just Don't Faint." Please understand the Lord called me to this, and I answered the call.

Spring was quickly coming to an end, and summer was about to make its grand entrance. I absolutely loved this season of my life. June is a month of celebration for me; from my birthday at the beginning of the month, to the start of summer, typically my vacation month, this was my month! As always, I took the time to do all the tedious things that I had to do, so I could get on to the fun things I wanted to do. I made appointments to have all my annual exams, eye, dental, and physical completed. This would be routine as always; so, I thought. During my physical, I asked the doctor to feel a particular area in my left breast. Due to having fiber strands in my breast, it was not abnormal to feel something, however, this seemed a little more formed than anything I had felt before. I discovered the lump during a self-exam, but I wanted to know if the doctor felt it, too. Growing up and being raised by a grandmother we were taught not to touch our body parts. It was considered "playing with yourself". And that was nasty. Let me encourage you to get to know your body. Examine, touch, feel, and massage it, so when something appears today that was not there yesterday, you are keenly aware.

Following the exam, my doctor told me she didn't see any reason for concern; however, she would make a referral for a mammogram, just to be safe. Safe was good right? Upon attempting to have the mammogram scheduled, the insurance company decided I did not meet the criteria for them to pay for a mammogram. It was covered for women 50 or 40 years of age if they had a family history of breast cancer. Well, I did not fit the bill, I was only 32 years old, with no family history of breast cancer. I thank God for having a doctor willing to fight with me at that time to ensure I got an appointment. I was told scheduling was backed up, so be sure to answer the call when it comes through. During the first mammogram, I had no idea what to expect. I thought it was like a simple X-ray or ultrasound. Nobody told me they were going to lift my breast, put it between these two things (that I'll call paddles), and press a button to compress them together like pancakes. All the while you are told to hold your breath. Did I mention I had fiber strands in my breast? The tech kept apologizing while I was calling on Jesus and at least 11 of the 12 disciples. I have heard testimonies from other women who breeze right through a mammogram. That was not my testimony. I thought they were going to pull this thing off my chest wall–oh, what pain! As instructed, I answered the call. Well, the second doctor backed up the primary care physician and thought there was no need to worry. However just to err on the side of caution and be safe we are going to send you for a biopsy to rule out any possibility of missing anything. Again, safe was good right? Go see the scheduling coordinator, the schedule is booked for the next three months, but the doctor wants to get you in sooner, "I'll have to call them to have you added to the schedule, they will call you with a date and time, be sure to answer the call, when it comes through," he said. With the biopsy complete, the doctor explained that the procedure went well. Once again, he looked me in the eye and reassured me there was no reason for concern. The results will be back in three to four days, we will call you with the results. And he was 99% sure the lump was benign. Good, after the third doctor echoed the same thing, I was convinced I was safe. I left the office with a strut in my step. I was feeling confident about the outcome.

On Thursday evening, three days after the biopsy, I answered the call. "Hello. Hello," there was a deep voice on the other end, asking to speak with me. I recall my heart sinking within. Working in the medical field, I know for certain when it is good news, the nurse makes the call, and when it is not, the doctor makes the call. This was no different. The doctor informed me the test revealed the lump was malignant. Baron-Faust reports that "every three minutes a woman in the U.S. is diagnosed with breast cancer and every twelve minutes a woman dies from it." "Oh, my God, breast cancer," I said to myself slowly. The doctor went on to say time was of the essence. This was on Thursday. I was scheduled to report for surgery on Tuesday for a lumpectomy. He apologized, knowing this is not the call I was expecting. Once the lump was removed, we could move forward with the best form of treatment.

Overcome with fear, sadness, confusion, and every other emotion I could muster, I pushed the tears off my face. What do I do now? What do you do when life hands you a bucket of lemons, but you have no strength to squeeze, nor sugar to add, all you can supply is the water from your tears, yet you must find a way to make lemonade? I began to pray, I grabbed my 10-year-old daughter and held her as tight as I could, uncertain of how long I would be able to do this. I needed answers, real answers. God, from the time

116

you called me I had three years of preparation time with my leaders before ever mounting the pulpit. Now, less than three months after declaring your word before an august body of people, you called me to the battlefield to let me die of cancer. I answered the call, but boy did I feel like I should have just let the phone ring, or hung up the phone when I heard the voice. This could not be happening!

Now, with the daunting task of having to tell someone, this would require me to say the words out of my own mouth. This was during a time when there was a notion that if somebody had cancer it was a result of life choices: smoking, exposure, etc. Like the story in the bible, when the question was asked, who did sin? Well, I was trying to figure it out too. I never smoked. I maintained regular checkups. Where was this coming from? I'm not sure why I thought I should be exempt, but I did. I was a single, working mom at the time; raising three children ranging in age from 9-12, and two godchildren in college, Alicia, and Darrin. What do I say to my family? Not to mention my pastor and church family? I only had four days to get my affairs in order. I reached out to one of my best friends and shared the news. He came to my aid as always and allowed me to cry while he drove me to Asheville to sit down with his mother and ask her if she would consent to raise my daughter in the event that I did not survive this. She agreed without hesitation. This was a relief, now on to sharing the news with my pastor. One would have to know my pastor. She is always multitasking, even during conversations. I walked into her office, with her typical greeting "what's up Stac" (only she calls me that by the way). Looking up from whatever she was doing at the moment, she immediately noticed something different in my countenance and asked what was wrong. What is this look about? I said, "I have cancer…breast cancer." Snatching her glasses from her face she exclaimed, "what, how?" Pastor Caesar so eloquently reminded me that God was still in the healing business and as long as I had breath, I was still a candidate for a miracle. She inquired about how I felt. The Lord had given me supernatural strength and peace prior to telling her, so I was able to reassure her I would be ok. Pastor was scheduled to be out of town during my surgery, upon her return she gave me a book that she bought at an airport and said she thought it would be a blessing to me. I read the book. The book laid out specific instructions and guidance on everything I would see and experience upon my arrival for treatment. To this very day, I cannot recall the title of the book. Once I finished reading the book, I was never able to find it again. I am glad to serve a God, who provides everything I need, when I need it, to navigate in life. Although I was raised not to question or ask God why, there was no one else I could ask and get an answer from, so I asked God why? While driving down highway 70, heading to the cemetery where my parents are buried. I broke down in the car crying and asked God why he called me out here to die. The Lord spoke to me so clearly, "I will never allow you to preach another's testimony, and you shall not die but live and declare my works, because I called you and I sent you to be a witness in the earth realm that I am still the healer of cancer." I immediately turned my car around, pushed them tears off my face, and said, "Lord, as long as you go with me, I'll go!" No trip to the cemetery for me, I had my answer.

When the surgery was over and I came home from the hospital, the real work began. I was assigned an oncologist. It was determined that I would need radiation treatment. What would this entail? During simulation and daily treatment, it would be necessary to ensure that I would be in the exact same position every day relative to the machine delivering the treatment or doing the imaging. Body molds and head masks were constructed to ease the process of remaining still. Temporary skin marks and even tattoos were used to help with precise positioning to target the spot. I received thirty-three rounds of radiation at that time. This was the maximum amount of radiation allowed in a treatment regimen without causing harm. I can still remember my first appointment for treatment, one of my friends from the church, Dorothy McCall was there for support. Little did she know, I was trying to talk myself into not showing up for the appointment. Every part of me wanted to run in the opposite direction. She was on time for my appointment, and I was late. She never knew I only showed up because I knew she would be there, and I did not want to disappoint or embarrass her by not showing up. Trust me when I tell you, God is strategic in all that He does, and He provides what we need when we need it. God knew I needed an accountability partner at that very moment. Every week, showing up to the cancer center, dreading each visit while sitting in the waiting room at the cancer center waiting for the call over the intercom like "Stacey Holmes! Come on down, you're the next contestant on the Price is Right!" But this was not right. It was all wrong. I have never been one that liked having my name called. I enjoyed being in the background, doing the work behind the scenes and not risking the embarrassment that sometimes comes with the spotlight. When these people called my name, it meant I had "it." Looking around that spacious room, nobody looked like me. Instead, everyone in the room was old enough to be my grandmother or my great-grandmother. Daily, without fail, I got "the question." "So, what are you doing here, you're so young?" Oh boy, how I wished I could answer that question. In retrospect, after the initial shock, going for treatments was the hardest part. Patients arrived according to schedule and sat around in what I would equate to a great room with a hint of uneasiness in the air. In this room, I contemplated working on a puzzle. It was the infamous pastime. The thought of working on the puzzle after realizing some started puzzles and died before completing them was not easy. The puzzles were on a large table, and people arrived and picked up where the last person ended. I juggled the idea in my head. I would not accept the fact that I would be coming long enough to complete a 1000-piece puzzle let alone lose my battle before completion was not an option. Continuing in the process the task of getting undressed and crawling on the table unable to move, waiting for it to be over only to go home with the same markings on my chest was exceedingly difficult. The appearance of my skin in the treatment area began to change. As the treatment progressed, so did the side effects. There were days of sheer soreness, blistering of the skin, and the literal loss of flesh from the burns of the radiation. It became almost unbearable to touch, I had to solicit the help from my prayer partner to apply ointment to my burns as the skin would rub off in her very hands. This was just a hump in the process.

Eventually, the treatments ended. The bi-weekly appointments turned into monthly appointments, and this was good. Finally, I reached a point where I was six months cancer-free. Then a year! No more sitting and waiting for my name to be called in this sad game show. No more daily undressing for treatments and climbing onto a cold table, lying still in the same position waiting for the staff to administer the treatment, or dragging myself back across the parking lot afterward with very little to no energy remaining. No more treatments. Thank God! I was finally at the end of this journey. My oncologist, Dr. Charles, was so patient, kind, and honest. With his deep accent, he said, "Stacey you're the youngest patient I've ever had with this diagnosis, but it's ok. By the time you have to come back to see me I'll be near retirement."

Oh, the excitement of hitting the five-year benchmark, the first five years are typically the watchful years for cancer to return. I remained cancer-free. Continuing to have annual mammograms with extra strength pain medication on deck beforehand of course– all clear. Ecstatically, approaching year ten with no cancer found Hallelujah! The oncology appointment was confirmed cancer-free–everything looked good.

I was in year 14 of being cancer-free. It was my birthday, the holiday about which I am always most excited. I moved about throughout my day feeling great, music pumping in the car, sunroof open, the wind blowing through my purple hair. I stopped at a store to buy myself something for my birthday and my phone rang as usual on my birthday. The only difference was it was not the normal 5:00-6:00 a.m. birthday call, this was in the evening. It was my best friend on the other end, so of course, I answered, fussing about the late call, because as history would have it, we were committed to being the first one to call each other on birthdays. This was what my father did, he knew how important it was to me and kept it up. I noticed he did not cut me off from fussing as usual and there was a different tone in his voice. He said, "Stacey I got some sad news, they said I got cancer." "They who," I exclaimed! "The doctor," he said, "I have throat cancer." I was frozen in time. I gathered myself. Dropped my items and made my way to the car. He said, "I'm so sorry, by the way, happy birthday, I didn't forget." Speechless, I asked The Lord to give me the words to say because I knew firsthand what this process involved. I encouraged him to hang in there and he would get through this, and I would be there every step of the way. I drove to Asheville to lay my eyes on him, anoint him with oil and do the only thing I knew to do at the moment, and that was to pray with and for him. We talked about the various cancer terminologies that can be challenging to decipher. It was amazing how similar our journeys were. We were diagnosed with Type 2 diabetes—one of the side effects of the radiation treatment. We committed to finding something to laugh about every day, no matter what. Only, we could laugh about our chard skin. I would describe radiation treatment as putting meat on a grill with the flame too hot and it burns on the outside but is raw inside, yep that's radiation in the simplest form. While he is navigating through chemotherapy and radiation, I was quickly approaching the annual physical and the dreaded mammogram in June for year fifteen clearance.

I arrived at the appointment, completed the mammogram, and waited for the nurse to come and instruct me to get dressed because I was good to go. The nurse approached the waiting area and called my name and asked me to come to the back. She said the radiologist wanted more pictures. Ok, soon I would need more pain medication if this did not soon end. More pictures as requested and back to the room to wait for clearance. This time she came out and told me to get dressed, but not to leave. Now I was feeling a little uneasy because this looks all too familiar. I did as instructed. When informed that the radiologist wanted to see me it was not good, but if I was still cancer-free, I was good. The radiologist popped the images on the light and pointed out a lump in my left breast. With a look of astonishment, are you saying the cancer is back after fifteen years? How could this be, I did everything I was told, to prevent this from happening. He asked if I came alone. Which I did. I came routinely for the good news. He requested a biopsy which was performed the same day. I was asked to return in three days, with a suggestion to bring a support person with me. Bewilderment was an understatement; I was in the process of trying to support my best friend through cancer, so I did not have time to battle cancer.

I returned to the appointment alone because I am not speaking any of this out my mouth until I know exactly what was going on. When I saw the nurse with the nice little folder, they put together for you with all the care team information headed in my direction, things became real. The nurse called me to the back to share that the lump was malignant. It was not back from before, this was a different type of breast cancer in the same breast, but in a different location. This time I was diagnosed with estrogen receptive/progesterone receptive (ER/PR positive) Stage 2 breast cancer. Unlike 15 years ago, this time I did not cry when it was confirmed, I was calm to the point the nurse was concerned about my understanding of what I was just told and asked if there was anybody she could call for me. I replied, "No, I am ok, even in this, I trust God." I needed to talk to my family, so we could embark on this journey once again. I sat in the parking lot and called my best friend and inquired about how he was feeling following his treatment. I gently said, "Hi! Guess what these people said? I have breast cancer." He responded saying, "Stop playing, are you serious, you already had cancer."

"Hello, Mrs. Haywood, I'm calling to schedule an appointment with the surgeon to discuss your options and recommendations." Once again, the calls were coming, and I was answering the calls. My family was devastated at the news. I took comfort in the fact my children had reached adulthood although I was raising my great-nieces. Things were in place for them. Radiation was not an option for me this time. The Lord allowed me to have a surgeon that was a believer when she shared that she prays before each procedure. I could see His hand at work.

August arrived, it was time for surgery, I had to be there at 5:00 a.m. My aunt flew in to be by my side. My two maternal aunts would be with me to provide care, while my husband and girls were at work. They would step in after work. My support team was in place. Prior to my surgery, the hospital staff told me, "We do not know who you are, but you have so many people out in the waiting room there is no way all of them will be able to see you before your surgery." Mt. Calvary showed up not just in person, but also in prayer. It was about 5:30 a.m. I looked up and in walked Pastor Shirley Caesar. I asked everyone to leave the room so I could have a moment alone with my pastor, she was the closest I had to a mother and that was exactly what I needed in that space. I asked her if she thought I was making the right decision to have a double mastectomy. We discussed what the physicians' thoughts were. I saw a look of concern in her eyes I had never seen before. Then she responded, "you do whatever it takes for you to live." They peeped in to say the surgery team was ready, so the pastor had all of them gather around my bed as she prayed and gave the surgeons specific instructions to take care of me and allow The Lord to guide their hands during the procedure.

The surgery lasted a little over six hours. When I woke up, oh the pain, I had never experienced such pain in my life, even after multiple surgeries. I was told they were going to get me up to walk so I could go home. In the attempt to walk, I developed a migraine. No one told me morphine would do nothing for a migraine. The migraine headache was throwing all the vitals out of whack. There was no way I could go home to my family in that condition. My daughter stayed by my side and prayed for me throughout the night and the next morning I was discharged.

Things were difficult, I could not sleep in a bed for weeks. I could not shower, dress, or change bandages without assistance. My husband would take me downstairs if I desired, but I would have to stay there until he got home to get me upstairs. Medications were causing me to be delirious—I was crying about everything. I was experiencing anxiety, depression, sadness, you name it. All at the same time. It was rough. What was supposed to be four to six weeks of recovery and then six months until my final surgery for reconstruction, ended up becoming a five-year, grueling process. Everything from a collapse in my expanders, a loss of range of motion in my left arm, and a negative reaction to the chemotherapy drug, and we will not go into the mental, emotional, and financial toll this ordeal had on my life. Through it all, people continued to pray for me, and I kept believing that surely, God had a plan on this side or the other. My heart was fixed, and my mind was made up, that if He did not do it, it would not be done. To add insult to injury, the insurance company dropped my insurance before my final surgery. If only the chemotherapy drug that worked for me wasn't so expensive. America will provide free Narcan injections to a person overdosing on opioids, but will not provide free cancer-treating medication for those trying to live. Each injection cost about 15k, per injection. Something is wrong with this logic. There were some dark days, even days I was not certain I wanted to live and fight on another day, but God made me some promises that had not been fulfilled, so He would not let me die. My best friend was healed from cancer, and I am happy to report I now walk in total healing in my marriage, finances, mind, emotions, and body. Thank you, Jesus!

Often, I am asked how I did it. How did I survive? A faithful Jesus and a dedicated support system in place were vital. Family, friends, other survivors, and my care plan team were all important. These people ignited my faith. Jesus continued to heal me. Family reminded me of why I was fighting; friends cheered me on even when I got knocked down to get back up again. Survivors confirmed I could win the fight and my care plan team kept administering the punches. At my lowest, God kept whispering to me, 'I got you", and you are winning the fight. This was my key to survival.

Despite all that I have been through, and no matter what comes my way, The Lord continues to call me, and I will forever answer the call because I am committed to an eternal yes, even before knowing exactly what the call will require. I answered the call, yet He keeps calling.

My Quiet Storm
Harriett D. Reynolds

What is it like to be in a "quiet storm"? I can tell you from my own experience that a quiet storm can be a hard thing to live through. I don't always see one coming but somehow when I make it to the other side, I am stronger and wiser. The journey through my first quiet storm began years and years before I heard those words, "Harriett, you have breast cancer". I heard my doctor say those words on July 31, 2012. Did I hear her right? I couldn't have heard her say that I, Harriett Brown-Reynolds, have breast cancer. "Yes, doctor, I can come in for my consultation. No, not next week, I would rather come this week….I am bringing my sister with me. Yes, I can come in at 10:00."

I have always believed in the power of prayer. And I also strongly believed that I would never have anything like cancer invade my body. I would almost brag about or even feel sorry for those who didn't have "faith" enough to get healed or defeat conditions like cancer. But here it is….breast cancer! How did I get it? As far as I knew, no one in my family has ever had breast cancer. Funny thing is, with all the questions in my mind about "how" I never asked "why". In fact, there was even a sense of peace in my mind and heart about it. I wasn't scared or anxious about what life for me was going to be like. At that moment, I believed that cancer was not going to defeat me, define me, or dictate "how" I was going to live my life. I believed my previous encounters prepared me for this and that I would make it through this "quiet storm" too.

A Quiet Storm…

It was 1964 and I was seven years old. My dad was in the Navy, stationed at the naval base in Jacksonville, Florida. Our family lived in military housing, off-base, which was situated in a nice, quiet middle-class neighborhood. I was really excited about starting first grade at the neighborhood school. There was only one problem, I wasn't welcome at the neighborhood school because segregation was alive and well. I would have to take the city bus 20 miles from my home to the black neighborhood and elementary school. I heard my parents talking about what could happen if I integrated the school. Mom and dad were fighters and refused to send their 7-year-old to a school 20 miles away on a city bus. My parents decided that I would go to the neighborhood school. I was too young to fully understand the meaning of the cross that was burning in the field across from our house. Mom did her best to explain the situation to her 7-year-old daughter. She also told me that I will walk to school but I will be under FBI protection and that a black limousine would follow me everyday to school. Mom said I would be protected because I had a "praying mother" who called me by name. She said that she always trusted in the Lord, and she wouldn't stop now. When I arrived on my first day of school, I saw the angry faces of those hateful people and heard them yelling and screaming about keeping me, and people like me, out of "their" school.

I didn't know if God was real, but I trusted mom. Still, I had to know for sure if He was real, and if He would protect me. I walked outside and stood in our yard looking up at the sky. The sky was clear and I thought I could see into heaven if I really, really tried. I asked God if He was real? I asked Him if He would somehow let me know that I could trust Him like mom does. I walked around my yard looking up into the sky and then I felt a hand on my shoulder. I couldn't see His face, but I knew it was God and He was real. I never doubted His existence again. Over the years, my faith and trust in Him grew and grew. From that beautiful day in 1964, when the true and living God revealed himself to a seven-year-old little girl. I admit I was a little afraid but I walked through those doors like I was somebody. Mom said I was. And I believed her. Forty-eight years later, my first quiet storm had prepared me for my breast cancer journey.

July 2012... The Truth of the Matter

The truth is, I wasn't surprised because I felt the lump months and months before. I guess I knew even before the doctor told me. I was use to doing self-breast exams and I immediately knew that something wasn't right. I felt the lump, knew it was a lump, but I didn't want to deal with it at the time. I was in denial. But every time I felt it, I knew that someday I would have to face it— just not right now. To be honest, if it wasn't for my son and only child, Steven, I may have ignored it for a lot longer. You see, I am a diabetic, and I somehow bruised the side of my stomach. It was a very large bruise. And Steven, who notices everything, asked me about it. Of course, I tried to play it off, but he is just as stubborn as his mother and as bossy as my sister. He insisted that I go to the doctor immediately. I told him I would. I didn't, of course. One day, in his very proper Steven voice, he asked, "Mother, have you gone to the doctor yet?" I couldn't lie, and I confessed that I hadn't. He got quiet for a second and said, "Mom, I love you, but I will not call you again until you go to the doctor." What could I do? Out of the love of a mother for her son, I went to see my long-time PA, Karen Booth.

I met with Karen Booth, PA on July 10, 2012. She ordered my blood work and completed a full exam including my breast. She did not discuss a "lump" at that time but asked about my annual breast exam, which was overdue. Karen simply encouraged me to make an appointment immediately.

I was still in denial and told myself that there was no need to worry because all of my exams have come back normal. That was not the case with this one.

I have always dreaded the annual mammogram because it was painful and very uncomfortable. I dreaded getting undressed and sitting in the waiting room with nothing on but a flimsy robe. I hated that the technician adjusted my breast over and over just to get the right image for the Radiologist. Finally, it was over, and back to the waiting room, I went. I patiently waited because it usually took about 15 or so minutes for the technician to come back and tell me what I always heard before, "You are good Ms. Reynolds, see you next year". But not this time. I saw the look on the technician's face. The technician asked me to wait because the radiologist wanted to take some additional images. Naturally, I was concerned; this had never happened before–still in denial. The radiologist reviewed the images and after what seemed like forever, came back and said, "something has been detected in the images". The Radiologist didn't exactly say what he saw on the images, but that I would need to have a biopsy done on my right breast. He sent me out to the front desk, and they scheduled an appointment with a highly recommended oncologist and surgeon, Dr. Nancy Crowley.

A few days later, I drove to my appointment to see Dr. Crowley. Even though I had no idea what to expect as I sat in the examination room, I was very calm on the inside. Dr. Crowley finally came in and explained that a lump had been detected. She would have to do a biopsy to determine if the lump is benign or malignant. She told me that a long needle would be inserted into my breast and that it would be very uncomfortable. My heart and mind were racing, but I stayed calm, even after I saw how long the needle was. As promised, the exam was very uncomfortable, and I could feel the needle going into my body. Dr. Crowley completed the exam and said she will contact me in a few days with the results.

July 31, 2012

I will never ever forget July 31, 2012. My cell phone rang, and it was Dr. Crowley. She didn't waste time with small talk and went straight to the reason for her call. Dr. Crowley told me that the biopsy came back malignant…I was diagnosed with breast cancer. I was stunned. Dr. Crowley wanted me to come in for an appointment immediately but gave me the option of waiting a couple of days. The purpose of the appointment was to discuss the diagnosis, what it meant, and the treatment plan. I held back my tears and promised I would contact her office and make the appointment to come within a couple of days.

My next call was to my sister, Karen aka "K". She worked in the lab phone bank at Rex Hospital and her job was to give patients their lab results and information. She understood how I was feeling. There was no question that she would go to the appointment with me.

The very next day, I went to the airport to pick up my best friend that I had met in Sacramento, California over 24 years ago at that time. Annette came to visit me almost every year after I moved to North Carolina in 1995. We had plans to go to the beach or the mountains and of course shop until we dropped. She always made sure she had room in her suitcase for all the stuff she would take back. She was only going to stay a week, but I would be dealing with the appointment I had to make with Dr. Crowley and who knows what after that. I did not look forward to telling her why our plans would drastically change...breast cancer...I have breast cancer Annette.

I was also starting the Fall semester at Wake Technical Community College. I was looking forward to my English class, Drama Appreciation. After my diagnosis, family and friends encouraged me to drop out of school because I would be going through a lot, including my treatments. They thought it would be too much for me. I wouldn't hear of it! I was determined that no matter what, cancer was not going to stop me from going to school.

Doctor Crowley sat across from my sister and I and delivered the hard truth. I had Stage 2 cancer, which was quickly moving into Stage 3. *I sometimes wonder what would have happened if Steven hadn't insisted, I get checked out.*

Doctor Crowley explained that a lumpectomy would need to be done, along with having some of my lymph nodes removed. They would be examined, which will 100% confirm that I indeed had breast cancer. She gave me some time to process it, and after I thought about it and after a discussion with my sister, I agreed to have the lumpectomy. The surgery was scheduled for August 10th.

Dr. Crowley gave me all the pre-surgery instructions, and what to expect. Once again, I was very calm, too calm. In my mind, I was that little girl back in 1964 when I felt the hand of my loving Father on my shoulder. You got this Harriett...breast cancer will not defeat, define, or determine how you will live your life. I am a quiet storm! I went home and told Annette; she extended her visit to be with me for the surgery.

There was still one thing I had to do, and it would be harder than anything I have ever done. I had to tell Steven...deep breath, heavy sigh. Steven Anthony Reynolds had to be told and big tears welled up in my eyes. There was no way I could tell him over the phone. He was living and working in the DC area at the time. I had no choice but to head north in my car, so K, Annette, and I piled into my Hyundai Sonata and headed north. We didn't talk much during that long drive to Steven's house. We listened to lots of old school music, including Al Green, Luther Vandross, and Anita Baker.

Steven being Steven was naturally suspicious that something was up. I tried to convince him that Annette and I just wanted to go shopping in the big city. I believe Steven, like the three generations of women in his family (me, my mom and her mom), has the gift of discernment or a "knowing"; even those things that are hidden. I could see Steven studying me across the dinner table. He was watching me, so I tried to turn his attention towards K and Annette who did just what I did and acted as if nothing was wrong. We were all just there to see him and shop. On the second day, he finally said "Mother what's wrong. Why are you really here?" We gathered in the living room, and I told him that I have breast cancer and that I was scheduled to have surgery in a few days. Steven cried. He thanked me for not telling him over the phone. He called his store manager and told her that he was going back to North Carolina with his mother. They understood and even sent me flowers the day after my surgery.

The truth is, there was no other choice…my son was going to be by his mother's side and nothing and no one could change that. It made me understand that the Lord's love for me is even deeper than the love of a son for his mother. I know that Steven and I have a special bond because he was in fact a Gift from the Lord. You see, 29 years earlier, after seven years of marriage, it was determined that I would never have children. I remember my mother telling me to go into my prayer closet and just talk to the Lord. One morning, I went into my clothes closet, lay on the floor and cried before the Lord. I was reminded of the story of Hannah. I must have laid before the Lord for hours. One day, I heard Him say, "you are going to have a son next year and this is who he is going to be". Steven came the next year! Another quiet storm and a chapter in my life that helped prepare me for the journey called breast cancer.

The Journey…My Quiet Storm

Words cannot express how I felt on the day of the surgery. Even though I was still calm, there was a sense of dread…I didn't want to do this! It almost felt like I was going to a funeral.

Dr. Crowley was expecting me and would be performing the surgery at Duke Raleigh Hospital. When we arrived, I headed to pre-op, and they prepared me for surgery. Steven's longtime friend, Jen, met us in the waiting room and brought a very nice basket of food for him, K, and Annette. It made me smile knowing that they would be munching on pastries and cheese as I prepared to take the next step of my journey.

The entire procedure lasted all day. It was emotionally draining. Dr. Crowley talked to me before the surgery and explained what it would be like. She tried to make me feel comfortable, but her pre-surgery pep talk didn't help. After the surgery, Dr. Crowley came into the recovery room and gave me the diagnosis. She removed 19 lymph nodes and all 19 were cancerous. It was confirmed. I went home with a tube attached to my right breast.

Dr. Crowley did a thorough job of explaining what Stage 2 meant and the treatment plan. But what she didn't tell me was that my right breast would be A LOT smaller than my left. She didn't warn me about how the look and feel of my breast would be changed by the lumpectomy. She didn't mention that I would have a permanent scar from where the lump was removed. I would later compare myself to little Nemo from the movie Finding *Nemo* because one of his fins was noticeably smaller than the other. I was very self-conscious at first, but over time I chose not to be even though the size of my breast was very noticeable to other people. Like Nemo, I would just keep swimming through my quiet storm.

Having a tube hanging from my breast made me uncomfortable and it was hard to sleep. I was exhausted, and emotionally drained, and I had no appetite. It was hard for me to even look at food let alone eat it. I got word from my sister, my gatekeeper, that people at my job wanted to bring me soup, snacks, or a meal. It was very thoughtful of them, but the idea of having visitors come to my home and into my bedroom just didn't work for me. Plus, the people at my job knew that I was an extremely private person and rarely talked about my personal life. The only thing I asked for was my privacy. It may have seemed selfish because I knew they cared and had good intentions. The only thing I wanted to do was dwell in my Father's secret place for comfort and strength. I was in the midst of my quiet storm.

So, what's next? I met with the oncologist, Dr. Mark Yoffe, to discuss my chemotherapy treatments. My sister assured me that there wasn't a better Oncologist in the city. He told me that I would have treatments twice a week for 12 weeks and that each treatment would last about four hours. I asked a lot of questions about my chemo treatment, and he gave me all the clinical names for the "cocktail" that would be racing through my body. He explained that chemo was not technically a cure, but it would help prevent the cancer from returning and allow me to go into remission in the 5th year after my treatments. He also talked about a drug that I could take for 5 years. And of course, we talked about radiation. I was not convinced and I wanted no parts of chemo, drugs, or radiation. I talked to my family and my son was horrified that I did not want to do chemo or radiation treatments. I had done some research and there were "alternative" treatments that I could do. I didn't want that chemo cocktail in my body, but against my will I gave in.

I was to start my chemo treatments in September, but first I needed to have a "port". Dr. Yoffe explained that the port gets placed under the skin near your collarbone. A soft tube called a catheter would be connected to a large vein above my heart. The chemo medicine will flow through the port flow from the vein into my bloodstream. It would be a day surgery, and I would be under anesthesia. I was dreading the whole thing, plus anesthesia makes me very sick. On the day of the surgery, I was still thinking about backing out. My son called that morning to see how I was doing and to get an update on everything that was taking place. I told him no worries, all is well, and I was headed to the hospital to have the port inserted. He wished he could be with me but I was glad he wasn't. I needed to be alone and deal with what was a head of me without having to worry about him worrying about me.

The doctor came in and talked to me about the surgery and to reassure me that it was a very simple procedure and would be over before I knew it. The anesthesiologist also came in and told me that I would be completely out and wouldn't feel a thing. I told him that anesthesia always made me nauseated. The doctor had the nurses prepare and as always, I got sick and went out.

I woke up in recovery and felt the place where the port had been inserted...I could add another forever scar on my body thanks to cancer. It is interesting that the scars from a port are very recognizable. When I see a scar on people that looks a certain way, I know. When people have noticed my scar, they know it's a "chemo" scar.

I am not my hair...

No matter how many times I heard about it, and the different things you can do after hair loss, I was not prepared. I didn't know when it would happen, but I knew in my heart that it would. About two weeks after my first treatment I looked for signs. Eyebrows were still there, hair was still on my head, nothing on my pillow, and no hair in the sink. Maybe, just maybe, it will pass me by. It didn't.

That morning I was standing in the mirror, brushing my teeth, checking my eyebrows and my hair. I reached up to smooth my hair out and then it happened. It was like picking a small cotton ball from my head. I felt it in my hand, I looked at it and yes, it was my hair. I reached up again, and another patch of hair came out. It came out so easily. It came out from the roots. It came out and it came out and it came out. And I cried. After I dried my tears, I looked at myself in the mirror and tears welled up in my eyes again. I was almost bald on one side of my head. I called my sister. She heard from cancer patients every day about their hair loss and she knew that the only thing I would have left was a little "peach fuzz". She asked if I wanted to shave my head. I said yes. K came over and the next thing I saw was my perfectly shaved head. I have a small nicely shaped head, which helped a little. We went and looked at wigs, I tried them on and purchased one. I tried wearing it for a while but it wasn't for me. Hair was never my thing and wigs were

129

definitely not. One of the cancer support sessions I attended showed us how to tie and style scarves. I decided to try scarves instead. Mom passed away in 1999 and I was blessed to get many of her things including a beautiful collection of scarves. Why she had so many I don't know but I was grateful to have them. Overtime, I bought a few more and learned to tie them. I always matched my scarves to my outfits, and they made me feel comfortable. I rarely showed my bald head to the public but I felt good about myself. My sister is a picture nut and one day caught me without my scarf and decided to take my picture. She said I looked beautiful. That picture comes up whenever my friend Annette calls me. I have tried to get her to change it but she refuses— even after all these years. SMH.

Why is hair so important? I was never one to obsess over hair. Growing up, I suppose I had enough, but it was never that important to me. I especially was not concerned with the texture or how long it was. As long as it was combed and neat, nothing else mattered. Years later, I still feel the same way. I guess my point is that I was never one of those women where my hair was "Me". In other words, "I am not my hair". However, the day that I touched my hair, and it came out like cotton in my hands gave me an appreciation for what I had. Even though my hair has grown back, it was not the same. That old myth about the chemo aftermath, and that your hair will come back "curly" and longer was not true for me. In fact, the thin bald spot, on the top of my head, is a constant reminder of the after-effects of chemo. What is also a constant reminder are the looks I get when I notice someone, mostly women, looking at the very, very thin spot on the top of my head. I see the look that says, "girl you need to get some weave".

True story, while I was standing in line at Walmart, a woman came up to me and said, "you know there are things you can do to help with thin hair". She went on to tell me about some oils, lotions, and potions that I can use to eliminate the bald spots. On the inside, I was annoyed that she would even assume that I was ashamed or bothered about my bald spot. I decided not to enlighten her and just said thank you. The fact that I have been able to grow my hair back is part of my decree that even though cancer took my hair, it will not define me. I will wear my short thin hair as proudly as I can because I survived, and I could have lost a lot more than my hair. One last thing, I want to say to people who judge others because of their hair. When I was in boot camp, my drill sergeant had a saying that I will never forget. He said, "It's mind over matter. I don't mind and what you say don't matter". My hair doesn't define me, because I am a quiet storm!

I endured my chemo treatments for 12 long weeks. Every time I went to a treatment I would walk into the cancer center, check-in at the reception desk, check-in at the nurse's station, have my port examined and sometimes cleaned BEFORE I sat in the chemo chair. Once in the chair I would try to relax as the needle was inserted into my port and the chemo began to flow into my body. I always took something to read and of course my music. The center was kind enough to keep snacks and water for their patients. I was never hungry but I did appreciate the cold water.

They were wrong about me not going to school during my treatments. I was in school the entire time. The one thing that kept my mind occupied was school. I was taking an online course, Drama Appreciation, for the Fall semester. My son bought me an iPad along with a keyboard and I laid on my left side and typed my assignments. Even though I was in pain and nauseated most of the time, I didn't miss an assignment, quiz, or test. The drama we studied was Shakespeare's "Hamlet". With my iPad, I designed the stage and set for Hamlet. I gained a greater appreciation for theater and set design.

I experienced some very unusual complications from the treatment. It was now October, and I was about four weeks into my treatment. I was determined to work, and even though my body was weak, I went to work and left early on the days I had my treatment. My team had rallied behind me and kept things going. I was a manager of the Financial Stability Division, and the agency paid for me and my team to attend a two-day housing conference in Charlotte. I was looking forward to the conference. A couple of days before the conference I was not feeling well. What I didn't mention earlier in my story is that I was diagnosed with Type II diabetes and breast cancer at the same time. I lost both of my parents to the complications of diabetes. I knew all too well how serious diabetes is. I couldn't understand why I was feeling so funny. I had taken my insulin, along with my other medications, and ate a light breakfast. Something wasn't right but I just couldn't say what it was. All I know is that I had a hard time lifting my head from the pillow. I had to get it together because I couldn't miss the conference. I knew that I couldn't drive, so I did the only thing I knew to do. I asked my sister to drive me to Charlotte. She fussed at me and insisted that I stay home. Somehow, I convinced her that I would be fine, I just wasn't up to driving. After all, I was still taking my chemo treatments and it was physically exhausting. That did it. It made sense to her, and she agreed to drive me.

The drive-up was a blur, I was so sick. When we arrived, I struggled to get out of the car and with my sister's help, I checked into the hotel. I laid down in one of the beds, my sister took the other. It was a two-day conference and I never made it out of the bed or the room. My sister did everything she could to get me to leave and go home. I was determined to stay and make it down to at least one workshop. I never made it past the bathroom. I spent the entire two days in the room drifting in and out of consciousness. I actually felt the life in my body leaving me. My sister kept testing my blood sugar and it would not even register. We learned later that my blood sugar levels were in the 600s. I was literally dying. The only thing I wanted to do was see my son. Just hang on Harriett. You have to see Steven. Finally, it was time to go, and I somehow made it down to the car. I don't remember much after I got into the car, I didn't even feel the car moving. I knew I was dying, but I was hanging on to see my son. Somewhere between Greensboro and Raleigh, my sister looked at me and said, "You know I am not taking you home". I tried to protest because I didn't want to go to her house. She had a dog. I didn't want to live with a dog. I remember trying to focus my eyes on her to protest but the only thing that came out was a very weak, "you're not". She said "no" and that's all I remember. Eventually, we pulled up in front of Blue Ridge Medical Center and she helped me into the building and into my PA's office. I was fading fast, but I heard my PA say, "we can have an ambulance take her across the street to the Rex Hospital emergency room or you can drive her". I protested and my sister agreed to drive me across the street, it took less than 5 minutes to pull up in front of the emergency entrance. I was admitted into the hospital once they found a room. My sister called Steven, and he was going to head to Raleigh as soon as he could. Just hold on Harriett, just hold on...Lord help me to hold on.

The next morning, Dr. Yoffe was sitting on a chair in front of me when I woke up. He was almost in tears. He explained that the combination of the chemo treatment and my diabetes was a lethal combination. He said that he would be changing my chemo medication and a diabetes specialist would be coming to talk to me about insulin, my diet, etc. He said he was so sorry and would come see me again tomorrow. Everything including him was a blur. I could not see him clearly and I just didn't think I would make it until tomorrow. When will Steven get here K? Tomorrow, Steven will be here tomorrow. I couldn't stay out of the bathroom, and it was discovered that I also had a very contagious condition called C-Def. Steven finally arrived and he had to cover up in the yellow hazmat outfit just to visit his mother. He covered up and I finally got to see my handsome son...the only thing that kept me alive. No, that's not completely true. I kept going and willed myself to stay alive not only because of Steven, but because I had too. I had to live because the treatment and now diabetes was not going to take my life. I am a quiet storm. A week later I walked out of that hospital and went home.

I returned to the cancer center for my "new" chemo cocktail. Chemo treatment was still making me sick. I didn't have an appetite and I was tired. I wanted to return to work full-time. Studying and being in school was keeping me sane. I still didn't want any visitors. I was just trying to get through this. On top of it all, I had a condition called Lymphoedema. I had to endure several weeks of rehabilitation sessions. I still feel the pain and suffer from Lymphoedema to this day. It is another constant reminder of my cancer journey. I am a quiet storm.

December 2012

Chemotherapy treatment was FINALLY over. Thank you, Jesus! I was bald, sick, and tired. The port was painful, but it wouldn't be removed for several weeks. The cancer beat just goes on and on. Thank God for my family, especially my sister. I wouldn't have made it without her. The semester was also over, and I passed with a great big A! I sent my teacher an email and finally told her about my cancer. She emailed me back and was shocked that I made it through school without one excuse for not turning in assignments or missing any tests.

She said, "the excuses the other students had paled in comparison." I am so glad I stayed in school! In the midst of the quiet storm, I did it my way.

It's not over. I met with Doctor Yoffe again! He discussed Part II of my treatment, which was radiation! For some strange reason he seemed very excited about the treatment and acted like it was the cure-all. Which I knew was not true. Radiation does not cure cancer. He was looking at me as if I was supposed to be happy about radiation. I was not. I refused the treatment. He was very concerned and horrified. I am done with cancer treatments. I don't want to be burned to a crisp with radiation treatments. I read the horror stories and saw the pictures. On top of that, the treatment was EVERY single day–Monday through Friday! I had gone back to work to my full-time schedule and now you are telling me that I have to have radiation treatments in the middle of my day. No thank you! I decided to let my family know that I was NOT going to go through with the treatments. I had already told Dr. Yoffe, and he practically begged me to reconsider. I spoke to my son and let him know that mom is done! Steven was scared and didn't understand why I wouldn't do everything possible to FIGHT CANCER. I tried to tell him that radiation was not a cure, just a big money-making machine. His will to keep me alive beat mine. Steven convinced me to take the radiation treatment against my better judgment and my will.

What happened for the next 8 weeks is too graphic to even talk about. When the nurses say that they don't understand why the doctor is continuing with my treatments, you know it is bad. My body was burnt to a crisp from my front to my back. I was in constant pain and my skin couldn't be called or look like skin anymore. My sister convinced me to let her take pictures of my condition and she caught me at a weak moment. It is hard for me to even look at those pictures even today. Radiation treatment is barbaric, and I once again bare the scars on my body. I had endured and suffered more than I thought my body could. On the day of the last treatment, all the nurses and technicians gave me a hug.   One was even bold enough to tell me that she had never seen radiation do so much damage. I walked out of the treatment center for the last time. I never looked back, and I will never take another cancer treatment of any kind again.

I went back to work. I went back to school. I traveled and went on several cruises. But from 2013 until 2017, what I didn't do was go back to see my Oncologist.   I waited until the five-year mark to make my final appointment with Dr. Yoffe. He remembered me and was happy to see me. He started by telling me that there is a drug that I can take for 10 years. I stopped him right there. I asked if I technically was in remission? It has been 5 years. He said Yes. I thanked him and said I will not be back. I walked out of his office and never returned. I survived. Breast cancer did not define me, steal my life, or determine what my future would be like.

The best card I ever received was from Steven on March 20, 2013, just a few weeks after my last radiation treatment. It came in the mail, and I opened it up. The outside of the card was covered in a fine red glitter with a small crown at the top and placed over this very popular saying...

Keep Calm
And
Carry On
On the inside, it said, in my son's own handwriting....
You Kicked Cancers A___ ___!
I am so proud of you!
With all my love
~*Steven*~

I AM A QUIET STORM!

Don't Die In The Winter
Kelli McNeill-Wilhelm

He woke me up with a kiss on the top of my head and said, "Good morning beautiful," like he does every morning. This particular morning, he also whispered, "your hair is growing back". I smiled and gave him a hug and rolled over and went back to sleep. The date was May 29, 2014. I was at the end of my chemo treatments for breast cancer. I had one more treatment to go and then my family could get back to "normal". To say I was looking forward to it is a gross understatement…but let's rewind just a bit.

On December 24, 2013, I went in for my yearly mammogram. It was Christmas Eve. It was winter. I was forty-four years old. I had been getting mammograms since I was 35 due to my family history. My mother and her mother had both been diagnosed with breast cancer in their thirties. My Mother, Helen, is currently a 32-year breast cancer survivor. My Grandmother, Myrtle, was also a thirty-plus year survivor. I had two generations of women before me who knew how to fight. Unconsciously, there seemed to always be a gnawing in the back of my mind–a nipping suspicion that I too, might be handed that same challenge some day.

Getting my mammograms was always a "gift" to myself. It was always a convenient time to get it done, as I was already off work for the Christmas holidays. A couple days after the mammogram, I got a telephone call from the radiologist telling me I needed to come back in for further screenings. She scheduled my appointment for December 31, 2013. New Year's Eve. At that point in my life, my husband, Wayne, was two years into his first Pastorate. He was also working on completing his Doctor of Ministry degree. Our oldest daughter, Nikki, was about to give birth to our second granddaughter, Milyn. Our oldest son, Jordan, was finishing his first semester of college. Our two youngest children, Jada and Justin, were a Junior and Sophomore in High School. I was working full time in local government, driving 45 minutes to Chapel Hill two nights a week to complete courses to earn my Psychology degree from the University of North Carolina at Chapel Hill, and spending all of my spare time with my Granddaughter Aubri. I really could not fathom adding anything else to my plate. I went in for my second mammogram on New Year's Eve and later went to our Watch Night service where I was one of the speakers. Needless to say, I was heavily preoccupied. It would be a few more days before I went back to the doctor's office for the results.

On January 9, 2014, with my husband by my side, I heard those dreaded words, "You have breast cancer". It felt like all of the oxygen had been sucked out of the room. In a matter of a few seconds, I experienced myriad emotions: fear, disbelief, anger. I was scared of the unknown and what was to come. I couldn't believe that I had been delivered this generational fate. I was angry. So angry. I was angry at the woman who had given me the news. It was the first time I had ever seen her in my life. She didn't know me but she had the audacity to be giving me the kind of news that would throw my family off-kilter and draw us into a whirlpool of uncertainty. And truth be told, I was angry at God. Yes, me, the pastor's wife, was angry at God. The seasons were changing. It was winter.

I shed a few tears while sitting in that doctor's office. I dried them up before leaving that office. My husband and I drove home in silence. He held my hand the entire way. When we got home, we both kind of just stumbled around the house, not doing anything but staying busy at the same time. After we had been home for a few hours, my long-time friend Sandie just happened to stop by. I always thought we must have seemed a little off to her that night. We didn't mention the news to her. Wayne and I were both still processing what we had heard earlier. I don't think either of us was ready to say it out loud. So we didn't. It was winter.

The next couple weeks after the diagnosis moved at lightning speed. We learned that I had been diagnosed with Stage 1invasive ductal carcinoma in my left breast and that it was estrogen negative, progesterone negative and HER-2 negative. Triple Negative. The most aggressive kind of breast cancer. It is most often seen in Black Women. The treatment would be just as aggressive. A double mastectomy followed by eight rounds of chemotherapy. Even though the cancer was just diagnosed in one breast, I opted to have them both removed. We're being aggressive right? They were trying to kill me! It was winter.

My surgery was scheduled for January 31, 2014. It was my daughter's due date. It was an 8-hour surgery and it went off without a hitch. Recovery, however, was brutal. I was sent home looking like the bride of Frankenstein and feeling like I had been run over by a freight train. I had been cut from the center of my chest to under my armpit on both sides. I had tubes coming out of both my left and right side that were draining blood into two little bulbs. The blood had to be measured periodically to ensure that my body was healing properly. That task was taken on by my husband. The pain in my heart of watching him in the role of my caregiver, who now handled me like a porcelain doll, rather than my husband, whose physical touch always made me feel safe, secure, connected, sensual and cared for—in a different way, was almost unbearable. It was nothing compared to the unimaginable physical pain though. That pain was excruciating. So much so, I was unable to lay down in any position. I wasn't able to sleep in my bed so for two weeks, I slept on our couch that had reclining chairs. Wayne slept right alongside me–

waking me every few hours to give me my pain medication and antibiotics and emptying and measuring my bloody drainage bulbs. It was winter.

On February 28, 2014, I started the chemo treatments. It would be 4 rounds of Adriamycin and Cytoxan, which they called the "Red Devil ". Imagine that. I would then get 4 rounds of Taxol. The treatments were every two weeks and they were brutal. They took a physical toll on my body but they were also chipping away at me mentally. On March 20, 2014, the first day of spring, I called my Sister-in-law Tameka to come to my house to shave my head. The chemo had made it necessary. Cancer is the master of surprise. There really is no way around that. It shows up out of nowhere, when it wants to, where it wants to and how it wants to. From the moment it rears its ugly head, survivors are forced to take the defensive route. If one is not careful, they may find themselves in a state of hopelessness, despair, desperation and/or depression. I was headed there. I still so much wanted to be in control of something where this disease was concerned but I was not going to be able to do that on the hair front. How could I be when every time I got in the shower, hair was lost from EVERYWHERE? Hair from my arms, legs, head, eyelashes. It was washed right down the drain with the suds—everywhere. How could I be in control of when I lost my hair when every time I put my hands in it, I pulled out a patch? How could I possibly have been in control of when I lost my hair when every morning when I rose with the greatest of intentions, some of my hair stayed put on my pillow? How was I going to be the authority of when I lost my hair when the texture had changed and it was brittle as tumbleweed in the winter time? (OK I don't really know how tumbleweed feels in the wintertime but I'm pretty sure my hair was REALLY close). My answer to the above questions is that I was really not in control. Not of any of those things where my hair was concerned. For some women, hair is tied to so many things; sex appeal, power, image, personality, acceptance, etc. I never thought my hair strongly connected me to any of those things but now I had to come to grips with the reality that I wouldn't have any hair and how that would impact me and how I showed up in the world. The seasons were changing. It was winter y'all.

Although I couldn't control my hair loss, what I WAS in control of was how I was going to react to losing it. Cancer had pretty much been in control of a lot of my time since that January day but what it didn't control was my outlook on life. Cancer forced me to make a decision to cut my hair that day but what cancer was not in control of was who I called to come and cut it. Cancer had no idea that I would call Tameka to come do the honors. Cancer didn't know that she was in the top 5 when it came to my "Prayer Warriors" so it couldn't have any idea of what was to come. Cancer had no idea that as I heard the snip of the scissors around my ear, my mind would go back to all those times that my grandma and mama would tell me to hold that ear while they pulled a straightening comb through my hair for Easter service or back-to-school preparations. Cancer had no idea that while my curly locks were being cut, that somehow I would catch a whiff of those ghastly chemicals that they used to put in my hair when I was getting a "curly kit". Cancer was not in control when I felt a tug on one side of my head that reminded me of those summer days on the front porch when one of my cousins was giving me a fresh new "do" of braids and beads. And Cancer certainly was not in control of what would happen next. As I heard the clippers buzzing and shaving off my hair, I was overtaken with all of these thoughts and emotions. Tears that I had been fighting back for so many months trickled from my eyes unbeknownst to Tameka. She may have remained unaware had I not taken a deep breath and released a long, exasperating, barely audible sob. She turned the clippers off and before she said anything to me, she just started calling on the name of Jesus. He heard her and gave her the exact words that I needed to hear at that moment. She reminded me that Christians love to spout off cutesy cliché's like "what God has for me, it is for me". She reminded me that EVERYTHING He has for us is not always cute. Sometimes it comes in the form of horrific trials and tribulations that we must endure so that we are possibly able to help somebody else. When He gives us something that is not so cute and maybe something that nobody else wants, will we still praise Him? Is He still good? Is he still worthy? Do we still love Him? She then told me that losing my hair was an awful, dreadful thing but that I was so much more than just my hair. I was more significant than the strands that now littered my kitchen floor. She looked me dead in my eyes and told me with authority and in no uncertain terms that I was already HEALED and this hair was a small price to pay for that healing. And through it all, God still loves me. It was me, and not cancer, that was in control when I sucked it up, dried my eyes, looked her back in her eyes and said "OK. I'm ready." It was the first day of spring but I was smack dab in the middle of my winter.

Winter is a time when things get dismal and bleak. It's bone-chillingly cold. The daylight hours are shorter. Darkness settles in earlier. The warm oranges, yellows and browns of fall have faded into dull blues and dreary grays. Winter is not a time when things bloom. It's a time when trees, flowers, and grass withers and dies. It's murky, shadowy and dark. When things are not going well in our lives, it may feel like winter. When you've lost your job, when a loved one dies, when your trust has been violated, when a friendship ends, when your children (or you) make decisions that will have adverse effects for years to come, or when you've received a scary diagnosis from the doctor, it can feel like the dreariness of winter. Winter can be challenging. Winter may make you want to crawl in bed and just stay there until things get better. Worse yet, it could make you feel like just giving up and dying right in the middle of your struggles. I am here to rebuke those feelings of helplessness and to demand that you not die in your winter. During my treatment, I was encouraged by those very words from Evangelist Christina Mial. They were not directly to me but instead in a two-year old Facebook post that came across my memories at the exact time that I needed it. Evangelist Mial wrote about a conversation between her and her sister, Tiffany, where they talked about how the trees lose all their leaves in the wintertime but yet they remain standing tall and waiting because they know their leaves will come back. They don't know when but they know they will. She challenged her readers to be like the trees in the middle of winter; remain tall and trust God. She went on to say that "not only do they wait but they are in POSITION to receive. They have their arms {limbs} stretched up high and their hands {branches} spread wide for their blessing to have room to come." Evangelist Mial challenged us to be like the trees for it is in our winter season that God can do some of his best work in us. It's in our winter season that He can use us to show the world that He is sovereign and that He still reigns. Our winter season is where our faith can be renewed. 1 Peter 5:10 says "And after you have suffered a little while, the God of all grace, who has called you to his eternal glory in Christ, will himself restore, confirm, strengthen, and establish you. (ESV). Note that it doesn't say IF you suffer but the Bible says AFTER YOU HAVE SUFFERED. With that in mind, don't just be any tree. Strive to be an Evergreen. Evergreens endure the same harsh elements as other trees during the winter but they don't lose their leaves or their color. They remain the same. Be an Evergreen. In other words, don't look like what you've been through.

As a woman, two of the things that differentiate us are our hair and our breasts. In the spring of 2014, I had neither but I kept my branches extended. Losing A LOT. Losing what felt like everything. Having days when it hurts to get out of bed but is also hurt to keep laying there. I got up and extended my branches and waved my leaves. Having conversations with God and telling him, "God I know this is not your Will for my life. You came that I might have life and have it more abundantly. This doesn't feel like an abundance God, but I trust you". I told Him, "you have allowed this to happen to me. Your word says by your stripes, I'm healed. I trust you God" but in my heart, there was ice. It was still winter. It was so easy to call my winter season an attack of the enemy. I think sometimes we give the devil too much credit. His job is to kill, steal and destroy. If he were a corporate employee, when it was time for his evaluation he would always get "meets expectation". He does exactly what he's supposed to do. Kill, steal, destroy – if you understand his mission, you can withstand the attack.

Just like the sunkissed, snow capped flower petals of plants that bloom too soon in winter, God always sends us a ray of hope. One of those rays was in the form of my AWESOME husband and Wingman, Wayne. I cannot say enough about him and how well he took care of my mind, body and spirit during this time. Everything I needed, he was that and more. I had to learn to let him be my caregiver. Even though it didn't feel sexy, his touches when he changed my bandages, held my hand during chemotherapy, or kissed my bald head nursed me back to health both physically and mentally. Even though it was hard, I appreciated him going with me to every Doctor's appointment and asking questions about my care and finding out what we should expect at every turn. winter was slowly dissipating. Spring was on the horizon.

Rays of hope kept shining through. Those rays came in the form of my family and friends who took time to check on us and to encourage us. Those rays came from an awesome church family at The Shepherd's Flock Baptist Church, who prayed for us and who allowed me to just be me even when I wasn't even sure of who that was from day to day. More rays came from the Sisters Network Triangle, NC, a National African American Breast Cancer Survivorship Organization. Their "Look Good, Feel Better" Initiative was instrumental in keeping my spirits and self-esteem lifted in those early months of diagnosis and treatment. Those rays also came from God himself in the form of an encouraging word to me through His many vessels. Words about pushing through and overcoming challenges were especially poignant to me during this time. If we never go through anything, how can we know that God is with us? If we've never dealt with addiction, how can we know that He is a Deliverer? If we've never been lonely, how can we know that He is a Comforter? If you've never felt weak, how can you know that He is our Rock? And if we've never been sick, how can we know that God is a Healer?

Just as the seasons change, so do our circumstances. I am eight years on the other side of my diagnosis. Because I know first-hand how fragile life is, I often take time to just enjoy the moment. I have a brand new perspective on what is important. I recently celebrated 16 years on my job with the local government. We now have four grandchildren. One of my absolute favorite pastimes is creating memories with them. Whether we are jet setting across the country because they said they want to see LA or just hanging out on my back deck making TikTok videos, I cherish every minute. My husband Wayne and I are now empty-nesters and will be celebrating 29 years of marriage this year. I very much enjoy all of the quality time we get to spend with each other. I feel so far removed from those early days of treatment when I didn't even want him to look at me to now looking in his eyes and knowing what unconditional love and adoration feels like. We are now 10 years into that first Pastorate ministry. I'm glad to be here to witness all the wonderful things that God is doing through His people in our congregation. I finished that Degree and graduated from my beloved University of North Carolina at Chapel Hill.

Some of us are headed into our winter. Some of us are in the middle of our winter. If that's where you are, just remember to dress for the elements, my cousin, Anita, reminded me. A thermal shirt to warm your heart; a toboggan to guard your thoughts; earmuffs to ward off negative self-talk; an effective pair of rainboots to protect your feet from getting stuck in the mud and being unable to move forward. Some of us are coming out of our winter. If that's where you are, keep pushing! Don't quit. There is Glory after adversity! Wherever you find yourself, don't die there. Don't die in your winter. Trees do what they are created to do without being reminded. How awesome would our life be if we did just what we were created to do without being reminded? Stand tall. Extend your branches. Assume the position. Don't die in the winter. Just like on that early May morning, my husband assured me that my hair was coming back, so shall your normalcy. Keep fighting. Spring will come. Spring does not mean that everything will be perfect. There may still be some remnants of winter. I still suffer with neuropathy in my fingers and toes from the chemotherapy. The neuropathy in my toes makes it challenging to wear most shoes. I've found great comfort in a pair of Crocs. My eyebrows never fully grew back. I've become pretty good at filling them in (some days). I still have those scars that go from the middle of my chest to under both armpits. They remind me that I am a fighter. I am a survivor. I am a thriver! Just like spring, there will be some agitations (pollen) and rainy days but if we stand in our purpose and keep moving forward, the reward will be greater than the setbacks. I'm so glad I kept fighting to live. It was a tough road but I wouldn't change anything that has made me the thankful and grateful person I am today. Keep clinging to His word ."For I know the plans I have for you,' declares the Lord, 'plans to prosper you and not to harm you, plans to give you a hope and a future."— Jeremiah 29:11. Don't Die In The Winter!

Back By Popular Demand
Kimberly Herrington

Count Me In!
Yes, I got it covered!
I will be there!
What's next!
Let's get this done!
How can I help?
What do you need me to do?

The above responses described my life. I was always on the scene living and enjoying life. Of course, I was that mom always cheering my son on and supporting the dreams of my beloved husband as I was living mine. I was always the "Career Woman", "Wife of the Year", and "Best Mom Awardee". See life before Cancer always found me pouring out, supporting others, and being present by popular demand. I enjoyed living this life. It was always fun, and exciting. And I always enjoyed the next opportunity. One can say, my heart guided my happiness and my life. Well, as we all know, sometimes things come into our lives to take us off the scene. These things may have people that were used to us now waiting for us. Well, that moment came into my life unexpectedly.

In 2017, I was diagnosed with Stage 2 ER+ invasive breast cancer. I underwent chemotherapy, and radiation. That diagnosis turned my world on its heels, leaving me wondering where to go from here. I recall saying, Why? What did I do wrong? How do I fix this? Will this be something I can manage? What will this mean for my family?

As black women, we always look at ourselves to be able to conquer the world. We have been conditioned to prove ourselves as worthy and capable; conquering all and never letting anyone see us sweat. We are accustomed to being the nurturer and caretaker to our loved ones and often minimize the value of self-care. And on that memorable day, when the doctor reviewed my report and spoke to me about my condition, I crumbled. Reflecting on my upbringing and assumed roles in life, I processed the impact of this responsibility on my health and my future. For far too long I had allowed myself to be a secondary factor in my own life.

I looked into the doctor's eyes as she spoke to me, but her voice faded and panic ensued. As my eyes filled with tears, my heart dropped to the pit of my stomach. I did not want to believe that this was happening. Although I personally knew women that made it through, I did not want to accept what

I was hearing. I was in a complete daze and did not realize all of what was happening. This was certainly something I had not prepared for. In that doctor's office, I could not stop the tears from flowing. My 45-minute appointment had turned into three hours. It led to meetings, consultations, and eventually a distress call to my husband. What had been a routine mammogram, prompted by my own self-check, had led to something that I had never fathomed. On this day, I knew I would never be the same.

Just a few years earlier, my mother had also been diagnosed with breast cancer and underwent a double mastectomy. Knowing what her experience had been, the pain she endured, and the physical and emotional battles she struggled with during and long after, I was determined to fight my best fight. We talked, cried, and even sat in silence during the initial phases because we both knew what was needed to rise above what has been put before me. During the experience of a series of appointments, tests, biopsies, care planning sessions, and research, I decided this diagnosis, this challenge that I have been faced with, will not be what defines me. I was determined to put myself in the position of understanding and trust in those that were put forth to treat and care for me.

I was very fortunate to have people in my life who love and care for me. People who have been there through all phases of my journey. Initially, I did not want to share my diagnosis, as I did not want to be pitied or burden others with my issues. It was even more difficult to share this news with my son, as I did not want him to worry and be distracted from his goals. At the same time I was diagnosed, my son was a senior in high school. He was in the midst of all the milestone activities associated with this accomplishment. While I knew there needed to be more focus on my health and upcoming surgery, I desperately wanted my son to have these experiences and transition to college without the cloud of my diagnosis hanging over him. From the date of diagnosis through my surgery, I relied heavily on my husband and mother to support me emotionally, and help me prepare my mind for the next phases.

Following my mastectomy, and subsequent surgical procedures due to complications, I started chemotherapy. These treatments tore away at my body—appointment after appointment. At some point, the feelings of despair began to fade. The crying spells began to be further and further apart. I began to look forward, look upward, and inward. Coming to terms with my body image was also something difficult to move through...seeing your body work so hard to fight the infection, change colors, burn, peel, and attempt to tolerate the pain is exhausting. I never thought that having a piece of me removed and the resulting transformation would make me feel self-conscious, inadequate, and even less than. There were so many pieces of my emotional being that needed comfort and encouragement that I turned to clinical

144

support and channeled my spiritual being/beliefs to rebuild my inner self. Unfortunately, at a time when having the support of family and friends may have helped, I shied away from those connections. It was too hard to go through constant inquiries about my experience. It was too raw. As time moved on, I had to develop a healthy balance and slowly re engage with my support team. After months of feeling as though I was gasping for air, I was finally able to decide that returning to some normalcy was what I needed to rebuild and to show up again. Eventually venturing into social activities and embracing the support of others. One of the hardest decisions I made was to return to work. I love my job, but I knew that it too had been a major source of stress that had the potential to place an undue strain on my recovery, but I moved forward. While working I followed through with radiation therapy daily for months. My life has been drastically different after cancer. My priorities have now shifted and I have given myself permission to pause and to put myself first. I can reflect on who I was then and who I am today and YES, I can say that my journey has given me the courage to make the shift.

Today I can say that this journey has allowed me to appreciate who I am, appreciate everyone in my life, and every experience that God puts before me. I have become more intentional about not holding back, and not being afraid to go for what I want and try everything. It is more clear now than ever that God's love for me is greater than anything that I know on this earth as he kept me. He held me. He comforted me through it all. He granted me the gifts of Peace and Strength. God reminded me that my purpose is to be able to share my journey; to help and encourage others and to be a blessing—as many have been for me. Life has many lessons for us… and my life lessons have been many. My life has not been perfect, but I know that my journey has taken me here for a divine reason…I am back! And back by popular demand! Remember:

1. It's ok to say No.
2. Living life on autopilot is not OK.
3. Yield, don't stop.
4. Never underestimate what gifts and purpose God has given you.
5. Today is not just another day, it's a day for you to shine.
6. Forgive yourself, It's ok.
7. We all have the ability to fight, it's up to you to decide when.
8. It's ok to be afraid, you're human. Be honest about your fears and be willing to face them.

Lights, Camera, Action
Linda Mahoney

Someone once described me as the epitome of the Virtuous Women. I guess I was raised right to get such a high honor. However, I held on to that as a valuable jewel. The mere fact that someone thought that highly of me, forced me to ensure I walked the walk and talked the talk. Therefore, all through my life, I always tried to treat people with respect, be courteous, and always share the goodness of God with them.

My life was always filled with lots of joy and excitement. See, I was a manager of a performance group that performed hits from the Temptations to Michael Jackson. This group of men became my brothers and my sons. Every week, we would travel from city to city and state to state bringing joy to so many. I was so humbled these men allowed me to work with them. I tell you, I had the greatest time witnessing lives being transformed by the performing arts.

Not only did the group have a chance to be in front of the camera. I was also able to be a hometown celebrity. I was able to play the role of a doctor in the public service commercial for the Children's Hospital, and three commercials for the SC Lottery System. And my days as a model are captured in the photo shoot with Augusta University. The performing arts was my place of excitement. Each time the words, "ACTION" or "Pose for the camera" were yelled, I became whoever I needed to be to ensure the audience received the excitement and joy. I tell you, this was a life worth living.

Well, as you would have it, life has a way of trying to dim the studio lights. In 2009, while performing my monthly self-check breast exam, I found two small lumps. I instantly made contact with my provider to assess what was going on.

When I arrived, I shared what I found. They completed a mammogram, but to my surprise, the first one did not reveal any lumps. We repeated the process. This time, they appeared. We also completed a biopsy. A few days later, my doctor called me into the office. Well, as we all know, they want to give you bad news face to face and good news over the phone. I instantly spent time with my savior, Jesus Christ, and submitted to his will—that it be done. When I arrived for my appointment, my doctor shared that I had Invasive Ductal Breast Cancer. I asked him when we could get this taken care of, because I had things to do and people depending on me. He discussed my treatment regimen and when we would start.

Well, I knew I needed a support system to help me get through this. I scheduled three meetings. The first was with my son and his father, the second was with my girlfriends, and the last one was with my family. Being the person I am, I did a "Lights, Camera, Action" meeting with my girlfriends.

I invited all of them out to eat dinner. And as we ate, laughed, and talked, I looked at the joy on their faces and how grateful I was to have this group of women. Well, I got their attention and told them I had something to share with them. However, there were to be no tears, they needed to listen to my instructions. As I told them my diagnosis, I also provided them with a call to action. I gave each one an index card with their numbers. I asked that they trade numbers, start a group text and work among themselves and develop their system of care. This was a time that I needed them the most and wanted them to lead the cavalry. They all looked at me with surprised looks as I stared back at them with a smile. I wanted to show them my love, and demonstrate my faith. Once my son was good, my girlfriends had their assignments, and with my family together, I was ready for the journey.

My treatment consisted of a mastectomy and reconstructive surgery. With the help of God and my family and friends, my recovery was successful. However, I still understand the importance of support. Therefore, I connected with the Cancer Support Group and developed a bond with the other ladies. We are still friends to this day.

Today, I no longer manage the group and have not been as active in front of the camera. However, after my journey, I embraced another stage. My moments of Lights, Camera, and Action are now giving hope to other women who are facing challenging times.

The year is 2022 and I have been cancer-free since June 2009. I am so blessed, and I know that God has a reason for me being here. I know that my journey was not for me, but it was for other women. I have been able to support so many women on their journey. And this is where my joy comes from. I also realized that it was my steadfast faith in God and his will for my life that has kept me.

Ladies, regardless of what is going on and where you are in your journey, take time and pose for God's Camera.

My Story
Angela S. Ashley

Greetings in the name of Jesus Christ, my Lord, and Savior. I am Angela S. Ashley, born September 19, 1955, in Gastonia, N.C. I am married to Rev. Charles L. Ashley, Sr.; we reside in Gastonia, North Carolina. We are the parents of Litisha D. Ashley and Charles L. Ashley, Jr. I prefer Psalms 23 as my favorite scripture because, during my ordeal as a two-time- cancer survivor, this passage gave me strength and courage to continue trusting and believing that God is my Shepherd, and I shall not want. I maintained my faith and confidence that God would heal me.

After graduating from Hunter Huss High, Gastonia, N.C., I chose Early Childhood Education as my field of endeavor; I attended Gaston College, Dallas N.C., where I received a certification to teach Head Start.

My favorite and fun things I enjoy are home interior decorating, cooking, exercising, and listening to music. Some of my fun facts are having a sense of humor and a willingness to laugh. Because laughter is the best medicine. It is good for the soul.

I have served as the First Lady of Galilee Baptist Church, York, South Carolina, for twenty-five years. This has allowed me to share my story of having survived breast cancer twice in my life. Upon arrival at Galilee Baptist Church, I was in the process of receiving radiation treatment. Many members of Galilee Baptist Church were surprised to know that I was going through a battle with breast cancer. My faith in God enables me to share my story and how I was able to be persistent in continually attending worship services and church activities during the time I was taking treatment. This served as a support factor for those going through similar situations. Being able to voice my dilemma and predicament helped many face the enigma and complications of dealing with cancer.

I am still active in church activities, Sunday School, counseling, and Children's Bible Study with Arts and Crafts. I am also working with vacation bible school assistants; supervising activities that support fellowship and hospitality for members, guests, and visitors.

I have had the privilege of being part of a television commercial for breast cancer awareness. CaroMont Regional Medical Center, Gastonia, North Carolina provided this opportunity to sponsor me as one of the selected participants to share my story with the community of Gaston County.

Before I was diagnosed with breast cancer, I was energetic, active, and vibrant as a homemaker who loved life. Let me tell my story.

In November 1998, I received a mammogram that gave concern; the physician ordered a second mammogram for more specification, which resulted inclusively. I will never forget December 25th, 1998. My family and I suffered a house fire, and we had to be displaced to a hotel. Two days after the fire had destroyed our home, I awoke with blood coming from my left breast. It was apparent something was wrong. The next day I visited my family physician, who recommended that I should see a specialist who performed a biopsy. The biopsy showed that it was positive for cancer (Stage zero). I felt that it would be cancerous because God had revealed this to me. In reality, no one wants to hear the word "cancer." In February 1999, the procedure to remove my left breast was followed by twenty-eight days of radiation. I am grateful to my husband, my brother Apostle James L. Setzer, Sr., and his late wife Clista B. Setzer for their tremendous, excellent support in doing this ordeal. I elected to have my right breast removed in July 1999 for fear of having to reduplicate this act over again. Unfortunately, five years later in 2005, I had a recurrence of cancer in my left chest cavity, and it was Stage 2. Therefore, in March 2005, I had to undergo surgery to remove cancer in the chest cavity. I began receiving chemotherapy in April 2005, which was extended through August 9, 2005. Also, I received Herceptin (cancer treatment) intravenously for one year following chemotherapy. This year (January 2022), I was able to be relieved of Arimidex after seventeen years.

After learning about my diagnosis, at first, it was deflating, disheartening, and defeating. I asked myself, "Lord, why me?" I realized that I was no different than anyone else. I thought about the hardships that Job had to endure. How he suffered, but he continued to trust in God. While going through this conflict, I recalled reading in the Bible in the Book of 1st Corinthians the tenth chapter, verse thirteenth, "There hath no temptation taken you, but such as is common to man: but God is faithful, who will not suffer you to be tempted above that ye are able; but will with the temptation also make a way to escape, that ye may be able to bear it." (KJV).

I was devastated when I was first informed of my first bout with breast cancer, but I relied upon my faith in God. My husband, Pastor Ashley, was the first to know what I was facing. Secondly, my children were informed. My immediate family was my biggest support group. They were with me every step of the way. I am so thankful to God that we all believed in prayer. It was tough and challenging, but God enabled me to withstand what I had to go through with God by my side and a praying family and friends.

The questions, "What is taking place with me at this moment?" I thank God that I am cancer-free and a two-time cancer survivor. I still have a solid personal spirituality of faith in God. I refuse to look back and ask why me God but look forward and thank God that he never left my side; I was a fighter who refused to give up.

"What are some of the words of hope" I prefer to quote Louisa May Alcott, **"I am not afraid of storms for I am learning how to sail my ship. We can't direct the wind, but you can adjust the sails."** I personally feel for me to reach my destination, I chose to fight for my life because I am a woman of beauty and a survivor.

The Conqueror Has Come
Willene "Thomasena" Wactor Brisbone

I can tell the world, yes, about this,
I can tell the nations, yes, that I'm blessed.
Tell 'em what my Lord has done,
Tell 'em that the conqueror has come,
And he brought joy, joy, joy to my soul.

As I have journeyed through life, the lyrics of the traditional gospel song, "I Can Tell The World" has always gotten me through some of the toughest times. For you see, no matter what life brings me, I always rejoiced in the joy of the Lord. For I realized that the joy of the Lord has been and will continue to be my strength.

My life was always filled with God, family, friends, and fun! Love is my superpower! I love people so much! I love to see them happy and enjoying life. Not a day goes by that I do not rejoice in the Lord and spend time with my family and friends. I enjoy going to church, singing in the choir, serving in the Women's Missionary Society, taking trips with my friends, and just enjoying life. Each day I wake up, I find something to do. This was my life before breast cancer. I was always on the move! However, life has a way of sending tests that will try to steal your joy. Well, my first test was to complete back surgery. On December 27, 2021, I gave God praises for the completion of successful back surgery. I was smiling, walking, and enjoying life. And when the new year came in, I entered it with a bang. Praising God, singing, and spending time with my family. For you see, family time is an extremely big part of my life. My family always comes together. Regardless of what is going on, you will find us eating, laughing, talking, dancing, and just having a good time. I tell you the start of the new year was great for me. My back was doing fine and I was feeling fine!

As life would have it, another test came. I went to my annual mammogram as normal and I did not expect anything but good news. However, my initial mammogram results were abnormal. Surely, it could not be cancer. This was the last thing on my mind. See, I lost my second sister to an aggressive Stage Breast Cancer, and my desire for the family was not to endure this again. Well, a week later, on February 8, 2022, I went back for a second mammogram and an ultrasound. Time passed and I waited for the results. Again, I thought to myself, surely it could not be cancer. Though cancer had attacked my family before, I was confident that I would not have to take this journey. Well, life has a way of trying you in the fire. I received a call from my doctor, and he confirmed a diagnosis of Stage 1 Breast Cancer.

Hearing this news, the only thing I did was focus on Psalm 46:10. I stood still and knew that he was God. Though my health was being challenged and my faith was being tried in the fire, I knew I had to trust his words. Therefore, I did not cry. Instead, I worshiped God. I inquired with my doctor regarding the next steps and petitioned my God for total healing. Well, my doctor shared that my treatment regimen would include surgery and radiation. And my God reminded me that he is a great physician. At times, the pain would cut like a knife. And in those moments, I worshiped God. When the enemy told me to give up, I fought harder. See, I had a reason to live! I had my God, my family, my friends, and my destiny. There was NO STOPPING for me! See, I had to live out the words of the traditional gospel song, "I Can Tell The World". And because I did not give up, I can tell you that the conqueror came to me, and he brought joy to my soul. Yes, that's right, after all I went through, I still have joy.

Today, when individuals encounter me, they see the joy I have and are often confused. They inquire "How". Well, my response demonstrates the regiment that I live by.

1. I had a support system. My family was there all the way. My church family at Mt. Olive AME Church, Woodrow, SC. My children were there: Lisa, Randy, Marcus, Renesha, Hermikia. They were there for me all the time. My daughter Lisa went to every appointment. And to say how good God is, she relocated back home without knowing that this would be a part of our journey together. See, God's timing is always the right time.

2. I understood the importance of connecting with someone that has walked the same journey. My niece, Tamara Wactor, was my praise walker, confidant, and friend. When I had a question, I would call her. She encouraged me.

3. I joined a support group. I am so grateful God connected me with Tamekia Hunter Ross and the Faith Strong, Inc., "BREASTies Support Group". Connecting with these women has been an amazing experience.

4. I continued to follow up on my health. It is important to complete your self-exams and annual mammograms. Engaging in your health is one of the key necessities to living. We are only promised one body on this side, and we must take care of it. Just as you get your car serviced, your body also needs routine maintenance. I thank God every day that I completed the needed steps on my health journey. Stay committed to your health.

5. Most of all my relationship with God. I believe in my favorite scripture, Philippians 4:13, "I can do all things through Jesus Christ

who strengthens me". Having a strong relationship with Jesus is the key to every situation, good or bad. It always yielded the best results. I believe that no matter what comes, I have Jesus inside of me and I can do all things but fail.

I know that this journey may not be easy for you. For my sisters or brothers who may be going through cancer now or in any challenging situation, please do not give up. I had Stage 1, but I know some of you may be dealing with 2, 3, or 4, but no matter what, DO NOT GIVE UP!

Today, I stand as a witness that the conqueror will come, and he will bring joy to your soul.

See You At The Finish Line
Bertha L. Johnson

Life can be alluded to as a "race or a "marathon." We must be readily prepared or willing to stay the course. Throughout my life, I always kept my shoes tied and participated in various marathons, 5K Walks, and other physically challenging events. At a young age, I started building my endurance. Walking daily was not only healthy; it prepared me for many of life's obstacles. Regardless of what the day brought, I always believed in staying the course. Well, as life would have it, the day came where I had to face an unforeseen barrier. This proved to be an arduous task, a marathon of another sort. Instead of my traditional experience with marathons, I found myself on a marathon to beat "Breast Cancer."

I was home in celebration of the Christmas and New Year holidays, 2016. Home for me is Upper Marlboro, MD. I'll never forget this bitter-sweet time. I conducted my monthly self-breast exam on January 5, 2017. To my surprise, I detected a lump in my left breast. The mass was very large. In my heart I knew the lump was likely cancer. Immediately, I phoned the breast doctor I'd seen for many years! She practiced within George Washington University Hospital Breast Center. I requested an emergency appointment. Fortunately, I was able to obtain an immediate appointment as I was scheduled to return to Texas the next day. During this appointment, my doctor examined my breast and ordered an immediate mammogram, ultrasound, and a biopsy. The doctor indicated based on her experience that cancer was likely, but confirmation was needed. The tests were ordered and executed the same day. The doctor also ordered an MRI. This was scheduled upon my return to Texas. On January 17, 2017, she called me to inform me that the results of the MRI confirmed cancer. This was the beginning of my journey to beat breast cancer. My race to the finish line had officially begun.

When I received the confirmation from the doctor, I was very calm. Afterall, I suspected the conclusive results of cancer. I mentioned that I was calm. However, I was filled with other emotions, not to mention the high number of questions. I turned my healing over to my Father, God. My questions included: Will I be able to continue with work? Who is going to take care of me and pay my bills?

I was a single lady with no family in Houston. Many of my connections in this area were from work. Beforehand, the awesome God we serve, placed a married couple in my life and we'd already become friends. The husband was a survivor of prostate cancer. This gracious couple saw me through the entire chemotherapy treatment stages. Without reservation they shuttled me to and from MD Anderson Cancer Center. The World-renowned center is located in Houston's Medical Center and is classified as the largest medical complex in the world.

My treatment regimen was Chemotherapy and Radiation. At the same time of my chemo treatment, I participated in a clinical trial testing a new chemo medication that could help others. I had Chemo treatments from February 2017 through July 2017 several times a week, transfusion for low potassium and magnesium levels, surgery to remove the cancer tissues from the breast area to include three lymph nodes on August 22, 2017, and reconstruction of breast surgery on both breasts. I had 33 straight days of radiation treatment after the surgery, October 2017 through November 2017.

My life after breast cancer is very different now. I am not as energetic and physically strong as I was before. I suffer with neuropathy (nerve damage) from the chemo treatment in both hands and feet, with numbness and tingling that sometimes affect my walking and writing mobility. During treatment the constant blood tests showed diabetes results that did not exist before. I now take medication for diabetes.

Though I have had a few challenges on my journey, I never gave up and that is the banner I always share with others. **NEVER GIVE UP TO THE SOUND OF CANCER**! Be strong and if you are not, be a believer in God to see you through this journey as no one else can. And remember, it is critical to have and keep a positive attitude; be around positive and encouraging people. DO NOT SIT AROUND, WORRY, BE INACTIVE and sentence yourself to death. I would also suggest that they join a support group, talk, and share what you are going through and take advantage of all programs available for cancer patients. I would also recommend participating in any Active Living after Cancer class.

To win my marathon, I firmly planted my feet in Faith. I maintained my belief in God and His ability to heal. Prayers were and remain important. I also refrained from listening to negative people with beliefs that cancer is a death sentence. Keeping this in mind is imperative while on this journey. Abiding by the orders from the medical team was paramount. My oncologist told me to continue living and doing all the things I normally do, and I did. Strength was sometimes a challenge but my ability to continue working was also major.

No matter what comes your way, continue to run the race. Though you may get tired, take a break! Ensuingly, tighten up the laces to your shoes. Continue your journey step-by-step. I'll be waiting to cheer you on as you cross "The Finish Line."

Young But Not Dumb…40 Saved My Life
Linda "Tyrice" Jefferson

No one ever told me that life would be easy. And no one ever told me that life will often throw you situations that would make you really ask God, "Where are you?". Well, my journey with life has had some good days and bad days, but I always found a reason to smile in the midst of those bad ones.

I always considered myself to be the "FUN" person. When you see me, get ready to laugh, cut up, trip out, and just have a good time. See, I was taught at an early age to not take life so seriously all the time. Instead, I was taught to laugh, spend time with family and friends, and do what you enjoy doing. Well, I did just that.

I grew up in a home where God was a priority; not an option. At an early age, I learned to call on the name of Jesus in the midst of any situation and to acknowledge him in all that I do. Well, I did just that. I always saw him as my guide.

Before there was a breast cancer diagnosis, you had "Tyrice", the fun spirit, loving, outgoing, big personality, well-rounded, and bubbly woman. I was active in my community. I enjoyed feeding the homeless and working with seniors and the elderly. I enjoyed my time with the seniors. For you see, they poured so much wisdom into me. And of course, spending time with my kids always brought me joy. You can say life for me was very sunny, with very few moments of rain. Well, as my grandmother would say, "Just keep on living". In 2008, some rain came into my life. Let's say it was more like a category 5 hurricane.

In 2008, I was doing my normal. I was smiling, spending time with family and friends, hanging with my kids, and just doing me. However, when the early summer hit, I was performing my "at-home" breast exam and felt a small lump on my right breast. Being in the Healthcare field, I knew the importance of getting checked out. Therefore, I instantly made my appointment but was told it was a cyst. It was explained to me that it happens sometimes to women in their 30s. I accepted that. I was in my 30s and living life, so of course, nothing like this could happen to me. Breast cancer was not even in my vocabulary during this time. However, something inside forced me to continue completing self-checks.

About one month later, the lump was still there. However, it had gotten a little larger. Again, being in healthcare, I instantly scheduled another appointment. I guess you could say, I believe in using my insurance. My doctor yet again shared it was a cyst. I inquired about a mammogram or an ultrasound. However, he informed me that because I didn't have a family history of breast cancer and I was under 40, the insurance company would not pay for the test. I felt a little disturbed at the coldness of his tone and the atmosphere of the room. When I inquired again, he said that I should not have anything to worry about and that because I am no longer having children, I will be ok. That did not sit well in my spirit. I reflected upon the words of my grandmother, "Just keep on living". Was this the storm that the prayers of my grandmother had prepared me for? I left the doctor's office with this large lump on my breast and no answers. Time continued to pass, and the lump got larger and larger. I could not sleep at night. My mind was always racing. I needed to do something. The professionals were not helping me, so I took matters into my own hands. I began to research and reached out to other healthcare providers in the area. And guess what, they all said the same thing, "You are under 40, have no family history, and your insurance would not cover the test". Now, here I am, a professional, hard-working woman, and I can't get a test done. During this time, I was still carrying this load alone. The lump was continuing to grow. And no one was helping me. As I mentioned earlier, this was a Category 5 Hurricane that was brewing!

As I continued to research, I was able to identify a practice that was performing FREE MAMMOGRAMS during breast Cancer Awareness Month. PAUSE...remember I said it was early summer and now here it is October.

I reached out to the coordinator of the event and shared with her what had happened. She inquired about my age. The Holy Spirit said, "Tell her you are 40". She said, "ok" and scheduled my appointment for the very next day.

Well, I felt it was time for me to tell someone. I did not want to go alone. I shared this information with the guy I was dating, and he happily agreed to go with me. I arrived at Franklin Square Hospital in Baltimore County. I was scared and nervous. I was filled with so many emotions I did not know what to do. Something inside of me confirmed I had breast cancer but needed to complete this process.

As I sat in the waiting room, I wanted to cry, but I could not. All I could do was hold my head up high. Well, they eventually called my name. As the mammogram was completed, the look on her face confirmed it. She looked into my eyes and shared she would have the pathologist review the test. As I sat in the room alone with the gold sterile machines and the posters of hope, I realized that no matter what, I had to fight.

Well, the pathologist and nurse returned. He told me that an ultrasound and biopsy would need to take place. When I told them I could come back next week, he looked at me extremely sternly and said, "No, you will need to complete the test immediately". I was connected with the nurse practitioner to complete my intake. From there I had to travel across the

160

hospital campus to the other wing. By this time, it was extremely late. I felt by the time I arrived they would tell me to come back tomorrow. Well, when I got there, they shared that the doctor was expecting me.

She walked me through my test results and some next steps. At that moment, I realized I had to be honest. I looked into her eyes with tears in mine and shared, "I am not 40. I told the intake person I was 40 because each time I tried to get connected for a mammogram, assessments, etc., I was told no because I was in my 30s". She smiled and said, "I don't care how old you are. The doctor does not care how old you are. The only people that will care is the insurance company, but today we are saving your life". At that moment, something broke inside of me. I realized that God had me the entire time. I realized that he never left me.

Well, by this time, my results were in. The pathologist shared with me she could not stage my cancer. There was a large thick gray matter which demonstrated being at stage 3–heading in the direction of stage 4. After that, she stated, "We are starting your treatment immediately". I looked down at my watch and it was now about 7:00 PM. I informed them I could come back, for surely the doctor would be off by now.

Well, to my surprise, she greeted me with a smile and said, "let's get started". She informed me that I would complete a series of tests to prepare me for treatment regimens. She noted I lived in DC and traveled 1 hr and 30 mins to be there. She offered to refer me to a provider in DC. However, I responded, "When I tried to get services, I was turned down. But you all opened your arms to me. This lump is ours together and we are going to treat it together. My life is in your hands".

My chemo treatment started 2-weeks later. My chemo treatment was doxorubicin (Adriamycin), better known as the "Red Devil". I had to complete 8 rounds of treatment–45 min each. The first time I took the treatment, I passed out. It was not because of the treatment itself but more due to my anxiety. They informed me I could go home and return tomorrow. My answer was, "No! I am going to push through this". And I did just that. I pushed through it. My friend at that time drove me and when he could not go, I drove myself. I was determined to live.

I had a mastectomy on the right side. When I wanted to do breast reconstruction, I was hit with another storm. While in the hospital recovering, test results yielded that I had Graves' disease, which turned out to be cancerous. Unfortunately, I could not do reconstruction. Well, I had to have my thyroid removed. Now my body was in a complete storm. I was dealing with breast cancer treatment and now treatment for my thyroid. I went back and forth to the hospital. Driving 1 hr and 30 mins both ways, in order for me to get the treatment I needed to live. Once the thyroid situation was under control, I was able to start radiation. For 34 days straight, I traveled for my 34 rounds of radiation. I never missed a beat. I just kept pushing.

Well, I still had not told any of my family. However, by this time, I was entering another summer. The kids were set to be out of school. I had planned for them to stay with their grandparents. I was not going to tell them because they were still dealing with the loss of their father with his journey with cancer and I did not want to scare them. However, with the final treatment, I would lose my hair. Therefore, I shared the news with them as a preventative measure. Surprisingly, they were strong. This time, I had another round of chemo treatment. This time it was Herceptin due to being diagnosed with HER2-Positive.

I endured the treatment pretty well. I had lost my hair, and would have some bad days with nausea. But overall things went well. After my hair loss, I cried, and I cried. As a matter of fact, I went and got a razor and chopped off what was remaining. My friend took me to the store for a wig. I found a wig and thought it looked really cute. I wore it for 2-days and after that, I could not take it anymore. Therefore, I just "Rocked My Bald Head". Now, everyone would know something was wrong. However, I had an aunt that wanted to care for me and show me support. This was hard for me because I was typically the caretaker and not the care receiver. After a few days of receiving care, I shared with my aunt that she could leave, but feel free to share the news of my journey with the family. See, I did not want a pity party, for I was enjoying LIVING!

Each time I went to treatment, God would not allow me to have a bad day. He showed me how blessed I was. While in treatment, I saw women that were on walkers, in wheelchairs, in canes, some were angry, and one had even lost her sight. And here I was driving myself to treatment and walking in with no concerns. I had to always stay positive and keep a focused mind. With a focused mind and halfway through my treatment, my hair started to grow back. My doctor responded in "admiration" of how well I was responding to treatment. After treatment, the continued test came. They found no more signs, or cells, nothing was left behind to even say I was knocking on the door of stage 4. Of course, I had to complete the five years of tamoxifen. I remained compliant and completed that journey.

I did not do the celebration like many other women. My celebration comes from when I meet random women on their journey, and I am able to provide them with hope. As a matter of fact, one day, I was on the metro sitting next to this younger lady who was crying uncontrollably. When I spoke with her, she shared she had just found out about her diagnosis, and she was only 24. At that moment, I was able to speak life into her, and today, years later, she is working on her master's degree, married with children, and living an awesome life. This is what gives me joy.

My journey was not for me. My journey was to let other women know that they can. I learned a few important lessons that I believe are the reasons I am here today.

1. Hold on to your spirituality
2. Be your own advocate
3. Don't stop going forward
4. If something does not sound right, RESEARCH!
5. Keep searching until you get the answer and satisfaction that you desire
6. Listen to your spirit
7. Do what you have to do

I realized that life means so much. Every day is not going to be a good day, but you have what you need to move forward. See, I still battle at times that I was not able to have the reconstructive surgery. I still have anxiety each time I have a mammogram. It is a constant reminder of my Category 5 Storm. However, I live the life I desire. Each day, I wake up, I thank God and ask him to keep my tongue in place. I love the day. I don't set an agenda. I just love to be a blessing to someone else. I have committed my life to doing something for someone every day. From feeding a homeless person to giving words of wisdom. I try to be a blessing to others.

14-years later, I stand healed, whole, and full of life. Out of everything, I realized I had to advocate for myself. The professionals were telling me no, the insurance company never gave me a chance, but I found a way to advocate for myself!

Still Shining This Little Light of Mine
Tamara Wactor

Living life to the fullest was always my story. I believe in letting my light shine wherever I am. From standing in the choir loft with my eyes towards Heaven and sending praises to my God, to just spending time with family and friends was the joy of my life or hanging out with my girlfriends. Born into a family of strong black women with strong faith, I had no room to run from life's challenges. As a matter of fact, I was that girl that dealt with the issue upfront and kept it moving. You can say that I was a modern-day Deborah from the Bible, the Judge that led Israel. Listen, with God on my side, a strong family line, and a steadfast attitude, I was conquering life. Each day I woke up, I always believed in making the best of it. I enjoyed going to church and singing in the choir. I can still remember Choir Anniversaries and how excited I was to wear my new blouse and skirt set with the other altos. On the 4th Sunday in May at 4:00 PM for many years, I would march in with the choir and loved seeing the excitement on the audience's faces as we sang our new songs. The joy that would fill my spirit is one that I can never explain. And more than 30 years later, I am still singing to the Glory of God.

Well, as life continued for me, I was blessed with two beautiful children, a girl, and a boy. They became my pride and joy. I live my entire life for them. Feeling them grow in my womb to seeing them grow into young adults has given me such great delight and joy. You would say that I had an amazing life. I felt that my life was a shining bright life. Well, as we all know, dark days often come when we least expect them. Well, when my dark day came, I was truly not prepared.

At the age of 33 years old, my life changed forever. I woke up to beautiful sunshine, but for some reason, I saw dark clouds and had this feeling of "something is off". Well, I shrugged my shoulders and kept pulling myself out of the bed to start my day. As I was preparing my shower, out of the blue something told me to check my breasts. I thought that was weird, but I proceeded with the check. And at this moment my heart dropped. As I completed the test, I felt a lump on my breast. Surely, this cannot be anything. For I am 33 years old, young, and thriving.

After my shower, I called a family member of mine and shared with her what I found. She instantly told me to make an appointment with my gynecologist. Well, I followed her instructions. When I spoke with my gynecologist, he said, "You have nothing to worry about, you are only 33 and too young to have Breast Cancer". Though I needed more to feel comfortable, he was the expert. Therefore, I accepted his statements and went home.

A couple of months passed and I noticed the lump was still there and it had gotten bigger. Well, I called my cousin again and shared it with her. She instructed me to request an ultrasound. I did just what she told me to do. The entire time I was nervous, scared, angry, and unclear as to what was going on. I had my children to worry about. I had my family to worry about. I eventually was able to get the ultrasound and other tests. I had to wait a couple of days for the results. That was the LONGEST wait in my life.

I eventually received the call from my doctor and he asked me to come in. the entire drive there, I reflected on my faith and worshiped God. I also thought of being born into a family of strong black women. When I arrived, I checked in. I was so nervous that I could not even write my name. As I sat in the reception area and waited, it felt like an eternity. I was able to use all of my five senses to experience the atmosphere and it brought me so much fear. Well, my time came, "Tamara Wactor, the doctor is ready to see you". I pulled myself out of the seat and got my mind together. I took a seat in the cold sterilized room and for the first time in my entire life, I was numb from the fear. My doctor looked at me and shared, "You have stage 3 INVASIVE Ductal Carcinoma". All, I could do at that moment was think about my children. Forget everything else, what about my children. Once I was able to get myself together, we started the discussion of treatment options. My regimen was going to be 21 rounds of Chemo and 12 rounds of radiation. Realizing I could not fight this battle alone, I informed my family. Of course, they prayed for me and with me.

The 21 rounds of chemo were the hardest. For you see, my chemo regimen was doxorubicin, or as called in the Breast Cancer World, THE RED DEVIL. During this treatment, I was at the lowest point of my life. For I always took pride in my appearance. However, during this time, I hated who I saw in the mirror. I lost my hair, and weight, and was often extremely sick. There were times I did not want to get out of bed. And when Radiation came, I was at the point of giving up. My little light was no longer shining bright. As a matter of fact, it was fading away.

I thought to myself, no man would ever want me in this condition. My self-esteem was broken and my faith was on trial. Each time I looked in the mirror, I hated the reflection. How did this happen to me? I was the woman that was living life to the fullest and now I am living life to survive. I found myself so tired one day, I was ready to just throw in the towel. I did not want to endure the pain. I did not want to continue treatment. I was just ready to let the sun go down in my life. However, out of nowhere, this flame started burning inside of me. It reminded me of my days as a choir member and the song "Use Me Lord" jumped in my spirit. And it all made sense at that moment. While in the choir, I would enjoy the words and how the spirit would move through the church as we sang this song to God's glory. And that moment, I remembered that in the words of the song, I told God that he could use me for his will. Instantly, I begin to worship God. As I continued to endure my treatment regiment, I was enduring it with my mind staying on Jesus. I prayed! I sang! I worship! I thought about being strong for my children. I thought about some of the ladies that started the journey with me, but they did not finish it on this side. I realized that God was sparing me for a reason and that was to commit to his will and testify on his behalf. My light was slowly beginning to shine again.

At the conclusion of my treatment, I had to rebuild myself...I had to get the oil for my light to shine brighter. Therefore, I took an entire year of work to get my mind, body, and spirit back on one accord. During this time, I assessed who I was. I gained my confidence back. I spent time with my children. And I returned to my love of signing in the choir. I now stand as a woman of greater faith. The darkness of Breast Cancer brought me into a light that is brighter than the one I had inside of me before. My faith is now much stronger. I stand bold on the fact that God still has me. I now live by faith and stand on his promises. Regardless of what comes my way, I now have a frame of mind that I will stay strong. I will not be easily broken! And I will not be afraid of what is to come. If I can beat Breast Cancer and endure the pain, there is NOTHING that will stop me.

Though I am in a better place now, I often think about what would have happened if I did not go back and speak with my doctor? What would have happened if I did not have my cousin to process this with? What would have happened if I did not have my faith. To answer those questions, I now realized because of 6 things, I am where I am today. I encourage everyone who is enduring Breast Cancer or who is now on the other side of it to apply these 6-things to their life.

1. Always maintain your faith in God.
2. Life is meant to be lived. Therefore, push yourself when you are ready to throw in the towel.
3. Focus on your reason to live. Mine is my kids. What is yours?
4. Always keep peace at the forefront of your mind.
5. You can be scared of something, but don't live in the fear of it.
6. You are not alone in this world. Develop strong connections with family & friends.
7. Communicate with your doctor and be willing to advocate for yourself.

After all of this was over, I realized I am a living testimony and if I beat chemo "Red Devil", I have the tools and techniques to beat anything that comes my way.

At 33 years old, just a young woman, Breast Cancer changed my life. The battle with low self-esteem, 21 rounds of chemo, 12 rounds of radiation, hair loss, body changes, depression, and the desire to give up almost killed my little light. However, I am grateful to say that despite all of the challenges, my light is shining brighter than ever. See, My God and I fought the battle together and we WON the WAR! And because of that, I will always **LET MY LIGHT SHINE!**

The Legacy Continues
Jean Bailey

I was born on August 11, 1937, to William and Mable Evans. At the time of my birth, African-American women did not give birth in hospitals, so I was born with the assistance of a midwife on Wade Avenue in Raleigh, NC. Since birth, I have spent my life in Raleigh. I graduated from J. W. Ligon High School in 1955. My class was the second graduating class from Ligon, as it was built in 1953 as the all-black high school in the city of Raleigh. I loved my time in high school and was the lead majorette for J. W. Ligon. This is also where I met my first husband and the father of my 4 children. My husband and I raised our 2 daughters and 2 sons together but later divorced in 1976. I was fortunate to have a career as an accounting clerk at D. H. Hill Library on the campus of North Carolina State University. I retired from that career in 1997.

I was blessed with good health for the majority of my life. In 1991 however, I was diagnosed with fibrocystic breast disorder, which meant that my breasts were more inclined to have lumps develop. Because of this condition, I had numerous biopsies, though all were determined to be benign. There was one lump that the doctors wanted to keep an eye on, and on June 23, 2008, following a needle biopsy, it was determined that I had breast cancer.

This may sound strange, but I immediately thanked God for the position He had placed me in to be able to fight this. I had remarried. This time to a dedicated and supportive husband. My children were all grown and settled and able to support me through the process. And I had a strong church family, with an established breast cancer support group that I could participate in. The first call I made on the way from the doctor's office was to one of my friends, who was already a member of that group. Her reassurance was invaluable. She reminded me of the power of God's love, and to trust in his will. The most overwhelming feeling through this process was trying to work through medical decisions with the doctors. At the time, everything seemed to come at such a high cost, and not just financially. It was recommended that I have a single breast mastectomy, to remove any infected breast tissue from my body. I agreed, but something kept weighing on me. I ultimately told the doctor that I wanted to have a double mastectomy. I know that God was urging me through that decision because it did end up that cancer was found in both breasts, and not just the right breast that it was initially confirmed in. After the surgery, I went through 8 weeks of chemo and 33 days of radiation. Praise be to God that outside of some superficial skin burns from radiation, I survived the treatment! I was confirmed to be in remission in November 2008, and have remained cancer-free since that time.

I credit my faith with helping me get through my breast cancer experience. I often read the book of Psalm, my favorite book of the Bible. Just hearing the cries and prayers that have withstood the tests of time, and applying them to my struggles, helped give me strength and peace. I also was determined to continue to live my life. I did not want to stop living out of fear or depression. I continued to host family Sunday dinners, and spent time with my great-grandchildren, creating memories. I believe that the purpose God has for our lives is always greater than any unfortunate circumstance we may find ourselves in.

Today, I remain a devoted mother to my four beautiful children, six grandchildren, and six great-grandchildren. I am an active member of Mount Peace Baptist Church, where I am a Mother of the Church, and participate in the Meals on Wheels Program. I am determined to live out the gratitude I have for my survival. I acknowledge that every day I am blessed to be: cancer-free.

The Philippians 4:13 Girl
Kimberly Curtis

I consider myself to be the "Philippians 4:13 Girl", I hold this scripture dear to my heart and walk in it daily. I attended Benjamin Banneker Academic High School in Washington, DC, and then attended my first year of college at the University of Pittsburgh, in Pittsburgh, PA. Later I pursued my Associate's Degree in Nursing at Prince George's Community College in Largo, MD, and later received my Bachelor of Science in Nursing at Phoenix University, in Phoenix, AZ. I enjoy bowling, baking, traveling, and spending time with my family. I am the mother/grandmother who loves her children and will deal with anyone who tries to hurt my babies (daughter 28, son 11, and three grandchildren 10, 6, and 5 years of age). I am an active member at McLean Bible Church where I serve on the finance committee and plan to join the welcoming committee soon. I am an active member of Chi Eta Phi Sorority Inc; Alpha Chapter. Our Motto is "Service for Humanity". We serve the homeless as well as the underprivileged and those who are in need. Chi Eta Phi provides health services, food, clothes, toiletries, gift cards, toys, etc. in and out of season during and outside of the holidays. Currently, I work as a Pediatric Nurse at Children's National Hospital during the day and by evening I am the proud owner of Kakes by Kim, LLC where I provide sweet treats of all sorts upon request. I enjoy serving people. More information regarding Kakes by Kim LLC can be found via Pop Up Events, Instagram, and Facebook.

I would have to say my life prior to my breast cancer diagnosis was pretty good, I was quiet, reserved, and more of an introvert. I remember getting my well-woman exams and mammogram screenings annually. With no family history, to my knowledge; I never expected anything to be wrong, **NEVER** expected a Breast Cancer diagnosis because I was covered by the Blood of Jesus. Well, April 2014 is when my life changed; I remember having my annual mammogram and feeling uncomfortable, I remember feeling the radiologist didn't know what he was doing. I got a call from the office a couple of days later informing me I had to return for more images, I then had to wait more days for the updated results, and then I was asked to come in to discuss what was then shocking news. I remember telling my husband "Honey there is no need for you to go, I am fine All Is Well". However, my daughter Kia wanted to go with me and man was I glad I said okay. The doctor entered the room and long story short started explaining the results, all I heard was **CANCER**! In the back of my mind, I asked myself "Why? What does this mean? What's next? Is this the end of my life? The doctor left the room and gave us some private time. I recall my daughter and me crying for about 20 minutes. After the tears, Kia said, "okay Hunni, as she affectionately calls me, I guess you will be joining the Life After Cancer Ministry (LAC)". LAC is a ministry that provides prayers, calls, visits, gift bags, and food when needed to those who are experiencing cancer directly or indirectly.

The doctor returned and I said "okay what now? What happens from this point? What are my options?" The doctor informed me that I had a diagnosis of Ductal Carcinoma In Situ (DCIS) in my Left Breast; she explained it was not invasive, and that it was localized and not found in any of my lymph nodes or other parts of my body. After explaining fully, the doctor gave her recommendation/suggestion for treatment; she stated a Left Lumpectomy, Radiation and Oral Hormonal Therapy (OHT) would be best for my diagnosis. She began to explain in more precise detail; I would have the surgery, after approximately 2 weeks of healing radiation would take place 5 days a week 30 minutes a day for the next 10-12 weeks followed by OHT Tamoxifen for the next 5 years. I left the clinic with Kia driving and I started making phone calls. I phoned my Husband, my favorite Aunt, my Parents, and a couple of other Cancer Survivors who are a part of the LAC Ministry; they formed my support system. The wheels in my head began to roll; so many questions and thoughts…. How would I look with 1 breast, how would I look now as a woman, would my breasts now be different sizes, would my husband still love me? **I WAS SCARED**! And then the treatment process began. I watched my breasts change right before my eyes, the left one turned black, it was smaller, it began to peel, and I even began experiencing pain in the left breast area. A little time had passed; It was advised that I no longer wear underwire bras and that I begin wearing camisoles. As a result of this experience with breast cancer to this day, I continue to wear camisoles for security. I continue to monitor and perform self-breast exams.

After surgery and radiation treatments were complete, I wanted to get started in the community I wanted to serve in whatever way I could. I remember vowing to walk in the Avon 39 Breast Cancer Walk for at least the next 10 years that followed. This experience opened the door for me to share my story on two separate (personal) occasions. First, I was asked to speak at an event that was hosted by a colorectal cancer survivor then I was asked my first year in the Avon Walk, May of 2015 to be the Speaker for the Closing Ceremony. At both events, I was afraid yet honored that I was chosen for such an assignment as this. I remember thinking "little ole me speaking before hundreds to thousands of people, wow what an honor". My coach from the Avon 39 Walk said she had never encountered anyone with the spirit and optimistic attitude that I possessed. I told her it was ONLY **GOD**, not me.

Currently, I am **CANCER FREE, PRAISE GOD**! I am working as I stated above as a Full-Time Pediatric Nurse and a Part-Time Baker and I enjoy both careers. Words of hope I would like to share and leave with someone is to surround yourself with positive people. Something very important I learned was that having a support system is VITAL! The root word "Vita" means **LIFE**, that support system becomes your LIFE line. Again, my faith in God and the scripture referenced at the beginning of my story, Phil 4:13, I now believe as an extrovert that **I CAN do ALL** things through Christ who gives me strength. I am a GRATEFUL Woman of God who believes and knows that GOD loves ME. HE chose ME because HE knew I could handle whatever HE allowed to come my way. As I view daily the scar that remains, I am encouraged and would like to encourage YOU, GOD IS JEHOVAH RAPHA, The God who heals. God has saved my life for a time such as this. Remember there is **LIFE AFTER CANCER**.

I Have Too Much To Do…So Trust The Process
Tomika L. Marks

My story started in December of 2017 when I went to the doctor for my annual women's checkups. My doctor asked me if I had just turned 40 in August? I answered her saying yes, I did and because I work at the hospital. She stated she would just put the order in the system for me to get my first mammogram done whenever I had time. I was at first upset with my doctor because we all know that during a woman's check-up with her doctor, they do a breast exam and she DID NOT find anything, but again she told me to be prepared to have my first mammogram done whenever I had the time to do it. Because I was a busy wife and mom of two active kids, I put off getting a mammogram for several months. It was not until February of 2018 I clearly heard the voice of God tell me to go get my mammogram done. I had a conversation with my supervisor and told her I was going to get my mammogram done. During my tests, the technician told me that because African American women tend to have denser breasts, I may have to come back for a 3D mammogram because something may show up, but that's just with African American women. And she wanted to let me know to not be worried if they called me back. I didn't think anything of it, but two weeks later I received a call and was told I needed to come back for a 3D mammogram because they thought they saw something, but again, not to worry because African American women tend to have dense breasts. I waited another two weeks and received another call and was told to come in to have an X-ray and biopsy done because they did see something in my left breast. At that point, I started to worry. They again told me not to worry because the spot that they saw was really small. Again another 2 1/2 weeks went by and now in the month of April, one morning as I was going to work, I received the phone call and was told, Mrs. Marks, you have breast cancer. At that moment my world stopped and all I could think about was not being there for my family. This couldn't be happening to me because I have too much to do. But I knew I had to trust the process

My life before breast cancer was one word ACTIVE with my kids. I was the team mom for every sport they participated in. I did not miss a game, practice, school activity or anything that pertained to my kids. I was diagnosed with triple-negative breast cancer, which is a very aggressive type of cancer among African American women. After having genetic testing, I had a lumpectomy. I needed to have two surgeries because after my first surgery they didn't get all the cancer out. My treatment plan included 16 rounds of chemotherapy. 4 rounds of AC, also known as the red devil and 12 rounds of

Taxol. Some of the reactions from chemotherapy was the total loss of all my hair, my fingernails and toenails turned black. I was nauseous all the time, and even my bones hurt. I had no energy. I did not have much of an appetite due to having thrush in my mouth and it hurt to eat. I had 21 rounds of radiation. That caused skin irritation and affected the range of motion in my left arm. I ended up having to do physical therapy to help move my left arm. During all of this my continued prayer to God was please allow me to be here for my family, because I don't have time for this.

My life after breast cancer is that I continue to deal with anxiety about any little pain I may have in my body. I don't have sensation in my left breast and very little in my right because of the reconstruction surgery I had. I was very thankful and continue to be grateful because I had tons of support from my husband, kids, mom, sister, brothers, aunts, and so many other family members, close friends, church members and coworkers. But If I start naming people, I will forget somebody (lol). They all stepped in in so many different ways. One specific person that I am SO grateful for is Lashawn Mobley, also a cancer survivor. We were introduced by a mutual friend. Because she had gone through the process, she let me call her anytime, day or night to cry with me and answer any cancer questions I may have had. I started sharing my journey on Facebook while I was going through treatment, and because of it, I again had support from all over and I continue to be grateful. Through telling my story on Facebook, I was also able to encourage other women to get their mammograms done and have been told that my story has helped several women as they went through the process. A few of the hashtags I used on Facebook were #faithfulfighter and **#trusttheprocess**. I knew that my faith was going to help me fight and that I HAD to trust the process that God was taking me through. On the last day of chemo, my theme song for the day was by Koryn Hawthorne "Won't He Do It". My life now after breast cancer is just always being aware of what's going on in my body and encouraging other women to get their mammograms and enjoying every minute I have with family and friends. I enjoy being a supportive wife and the active mom that I am. I continue to trust God's process with both of my kids who are in high school now and I have to see what they do. So I don't have time for any sickness.

Words of encouragement that I would give someone else that is going through breast cancer is to never give up and always stay positive; find your reason to live. You don't have time for cancer. I remember doing cancer treatments, I always said I don't have time to have cancer, I have too much to do. I have a husband and kids that need me so I need to get through this, so I can get back to what I was doing before breast cancer.

Free of Fear
Jennyveia K. Persaud

During the summer of 2020, amid the pandemic of COVID-19, I noticed that my left breast was slightly larger than the other one. Initially, I thought nothing of it. However, one day, while breastfeeding my then 2-year-old, I also noticed that she stopped gravitating to the same breast. I found that to be odd because that breast is the one she had become accustomed to falling asleep with. I asked my husband if he noticed a difference in size and he had not. I spoke with my mother regarding my claim and was advised to put a warm washcloth on it because it could simply be milk build-up from breastfeeding. After a few weeks, I got out of the shower and the breast was undeniably larger than the other. I stood in the mirror and gave myself a "self" breast examination. I massaged the cup and lo and behold, above the areola, there was a golf ball-sized mass. I still was not really concerned, because not in my wildest dreams did I think that the cause of my breast enlargement could be anything other than excess milk as I was a stay-at-home mom who has breastfed constantly for the past 34 months. Yet again, I attempted showers with hot compressions and to my surprise, a reduction in size did not occur. Once again, I asked my husband if he saw a difference in size, and this time he suggested that one was a bit fuller than the other. Therefore, I attempted to make an appointment with my primary care physician and was told that it would be 3 weeks before I could see her. When the day came for the appointment, I met with her and was somewhat assured that my theory of milk build-up was probably correct, but she sent me to get a mammogram to be on the "safe" side. Thing is, that appointment would be three and a half weeks after my primary care appointment. After the mammogram was administered, I was told to wait around to speak with the doctor about the images. A woman walked into the office and alluded to the possibility of it being cancerous due to the lump revealed by the photographs. She herself was a cancer survivor by way of a double mastectomy. Also, she disclosed that breast cancer is not seen as a death sentence anymore because of the scientific advances of the last 20 years. However, my diagnosis still had not been confirmed. Then, I was referred to have a biopsy and this appointment would be two weeks after my mammogram appointment. When the day came for my biopsy, I felt a bit concerned about what would be found, because my mammogram confirmed that I had four lumps beneath my breast and three lumps between the pit of my arm. Unlike the mammogram, the biopsy was a bit painful as they had to cut pieces of the 7 tumors the mammogram had revealed. After the appointment, I was unable to raise my arm due to these incisions. Three days later, I received a call from someone stating that I had a "mild" case of breast cancer. I could not believe how calm and unconcerned this guy sounded, whoever he was because he did not even care to disclose his credentials. I was told that my doctor was on vacation and to find an oncologist to help me determine what the next steps should be. I really did not know what to think at this point. Were they telling me that I was going to die? I notified my husband, and I could tell he too did not know what to make of this out-of-the-blue diagnosis. He tried not to show me he was worried and assured me that we would get through this no matter what. At that point, I do not think either one of us believed that. I located an oncologist within the same hospital and was referred for a pet scan (with contrast), cat scan, and a bone examination. He also referred me to a surgeon to speak with me about my options. Like the woman that gave me the biopsy results, the oncologist seemed like this was nothing he had not seen before and that the surgeon would provide me with the details of how they planned to proceed with eliminating the cancer. After the uncertainty of all the tests and scans I endured, it was time to meet with the surgeon to get some answers, options, and the TRUTH! My husband and I sat in the surgeon's office patiently waiting with so many questions that we both could not articulate. The surgeon entered the room upbeat, giving us the impression that she had some news that could change our outlook on our situation. She disclosed to us that I was currently Stage 2, which meant that an operation, by way of a mastectomy, would be part of their plan of action. However, I would have to take chemotherapy for a few months before the surgery and then undergo months of radiation to extinguish any cancer left over in my body. The surgeon mapped out exactly what this journey would look like and what we should anticipate at different stages of treatment. First, I would have to get a port put in my chest for them to pump the chemotherapy through my system. The idea of them cutting my chest open validated how real this truly was.

Once again, my husband and I went to the appointment praying everything would go as planned with little to no painful ramifications. After kissing my husband and he faithfully assuring me that everything would be okay, I walked into the room where the procedure would take place, more nervous than I was when I gave birth to my first child. Unbeknownst to me, they would have to not only cut into my chest, but an opening would have to be made in my neck for them to run the stem of the port through my juggler's vein. They monitored my heart throughout the procedure, and for a moment, my heart rate increased due to the reality of this whole ordeal beginning to set in my mind. There was a curtain in front of my face, so I could not see who was in the room, nor what was taking place. However, there was a West Indian nurse who sounded like my mother that calmed me down; helping me relax with her soft and supportive tone. After about an hour, the procedure was over. With a foreign object bulging out of my upper chest, I instantly felt like a cancer patient. The following week I was scheduled to begin chemotherapy. However, I received a phone call informing me that I should come in a few days earlier. I thought nothing of it but figured that a slot was open to start my treatment earlier. My husband usually accompanied me, but on this day, I told him to stay home with our daughters. I went to the appointment and was told to sit tight, and someone would be out to come to get me. Moreover, I was asked if I had come alone, which I thought was quite strange. Before I went to the appointment, I checked the *MyChart* portal to see if any results from my recent scan had come back. I noticed that they mentioned something about my liver but really could not understand the medical terms they were referring to. A few minutes later, a woman came out to get me and sat me in a room that resembled a lawyer's office. I waited a few more minutes before a male doctor walked into the office, immediately asking me how I felt. I assured him that I felt alright but inquired about why he asked. He took a deep breath and informed me that the scan had revealed that cancer in fact traveled to my liver and 10 lesions were the effects of my now Stage 4 diagnosis. I asked him what this meant? He took a longer and deeper breath and slowly said, "You have four to five years to live, and there's nothing more we can do". Was I dreaming? I was a month shy of my 34th birthday and was being told that I would not make it to my 40th. At this point, my daughters were just 8 and 3 years old. I broke down in hysteria and told them that I needed to call my husband. When he picked up the phone, I could barely speak. He screamed, "What's wrong, what's wrong?" But I could not reply. I passed the phone to the doctor, and he urged my husband to get here as quickly as he could. I sat there in silence for the next 10 minutes, thinking How did this happen? Why did this happen? Can my husband raise our two children alone?

My husband got there 10 minutes later and was escorted to the room I sat in shuddering. By the look on my face when he walked in, he could tell that something was WRONG! He asked me, "So what's going on?" I just looked up at the doctor and he proceeded to restate the worst news of my life. My husband emphatically asked, "So what are you saying?" The doctor rebutted, "There's nothing we can do, your wife has four years, five years tops to live." He went on to tell a story about a woman that had a comparable diagnosis that lived seven years, two years longer than they expected (as if that would be taken as good news to us at this point). He went on to inform us that there was a trial the hospital was administering where basically they used cancer patients as guinea pigs to study the effects of the medication. My husband and I sat there in silence for a minute or so and then my husband rose out of his chair and told the doctor that we would be getting another opinion and that their "trial" would be something that we would have to think about. My husband called his parents to drive our car home, as I was in a state of disbelief and disarray. At this point, I was taking the diagnosis of Stage 4 cancer as a death sentence because I had only heard the term used shortly before someone died from the disease.

For the next two days, my husband and I walked around in a daze, not knowing if what the doctor was saying would come to fruition. All I truly thought about was my 2 daughters and how this would impact their lives. Was it possible that I would not be present for my youngest daughter's first day of school? Would I be around to have the discussion with my eldest daughter about the process of developing into a woman? And my husband, whom I had been with for 15 years, would my diagnosis enable him to give in to the worldly demons he had recently conquered? After a few days, my husband showed me how much he truly loved me and would not allow me to wither away without a fight. He spoke to the doctor that gave us the news about the "trial" he mentioned in the hospital. My husband kept informing me that for some reason he did not have faith in this study and that something just did not seem right about the invitation. Therefore, my husband hit the ground running by researching and googling leading oncologists in the country. Lo and behold, he stumbled across Memorial Sloan Kettering (MSK). Unbeknownst to both of us at the time, (MSK) was the 2nd leading cancer center in America. We did not really know what finding this cancer center truly meant at the time because my Stage 4 diagnosis was presented as a death sentence. Like most people, we considered the credence of what a physician, who is a mere mortal such as ourselves, believes and most people take their word as "gospel". My husband reached out to (MSK) informing them of our situation and immediately we were transferred to their billing department. We did not know if health insurance covered cancer treatment or anything that came along with a road to "recovery". We were informed by the billing department that (MSK) did not take my insurance and they truly could not move forward before changing insurance providers. This was the first of many bumps in the road we encountered, but as I said, I noticed my husband's vigilance during this ordeal and he would not allow anything to stand in his way of putting us in a position for progression. Before the diagnosis, we had plans to move South for the betterment and quality of life of our family. It took us about three days to get in contact with someone that would articulate the process of changing insurance and how long this process would take. We were informed that the act of changing insurance was quite simple, but it would take a week or so for it to show up in the system and a month for me to get the actual insurance card. We consulted (MSK) and were basically told that they could not schedule a consultation with a physician before this member number was available. There were minutes in between these exchanges of "bad news" that we asked ourselves, "Why is this happening to us?" But contrary to popular belief, prayer pays dividends! Out of the blue, I was made aware by my cousin that her husband was employed by (MSK). Without having to ask, she notified me that he would be speaking to his comrades regarding our current dilemma and desire to expedite this process. We were provided a number to a woman that my husband spoke with (whom we later regarded as an angel in disguise). They discussed my situation in detail, disclosing the severity of the diagnosis, the preciousness of our children, the anguish this "bad dream" has caused our family, and more importantly, the acknowledgment of mortality by way of this deadly disease. When my husband disconnected the phone call, he had a tentatively convinced look on his face. As if things would start making sense. He informed me that the angelic soul he spoke with would allow us to provide her with all of the information the previous hospital had regarding me and my diagnosis. Moreover, we would have to also submit the images from all of the scans that were administered before and after my diagnosis. This was a breath of fresh air because finally, we were being given a path towards some type of answer and reasoning behind what I was facing.

The following morning, my husband got up bright and early to consult medical records to locate my documentation and internal images. He left numerous messages throughout the day, informing whoever would respond to our urgency. Later that afternoon, he tried one last time before "happy hour", desperately hoping that someone would answer the phone, and they did. A stern older woman answered and basically told him that usually, this request could take up to a week to be managed and met. Once again, he articulated the urgency of this request, but the woman informed him that there was another place he could contact to possibly get what he needed when he needed it. The very next morning we arose, thinking about what the medical representative informed him, but during this time, we both felt as though we were literally gasping for air every few minutes while drowning in the ocean. We took a deep breath and ventured to the address we were provided by the woman he spoke with in medical records. We drove over there, and the area looked like a ghost town, which we would soon find out that it was. This was 6 months after the onset of the Coronavirus. We entered the building and there stood a security guard shocked to see us. We asked what floor we could go to get what we needed and we were informed that the building was closed to the public for months now. Another roadblock stood before us! However, he mentioned that we could check the main clinic we had to go to anyway to get the slides that showed exactly where the cancer

181

was in my body. As we were getting our temperature checked, before entering, we heard someone mention "medical records" and gesture toward the right-wing of the hospital. We assumed that's where we were going to get the slides. We made haste towards the right-wing and hesitantly knocked on the door where an older woman sat gazing at her computer. My husband asked were we in the right place for the slides and she sternly said, "NO, I told you yesterday, where to go!" My husband responded, "Are you the woman I spoke with yesterday?" She totally ignored his question but insisted that we hurry up and go to the image center down the hallway and come right back here after we are done. We made our way to the image center, waited about 45 minutes for the images to be provided to us, and went straight back to the woman's office. It was now 4:30 pm and this was usually quitting time for the woman, but she was expecting and accepted us back into her office. By the sound of her voice and charisma, my husband was sure that this was the same woman from yesterday. We informed her that we went to the medical center across town, but they were closed. We disclosed my diagnosis and informed her that we were encouraged by MSK to also print ALL her medical records. She empathized with our story by sharing with us that she had lost her sister to cancer 2 years ago. Her sister was being treated, or so she assumed by an oncologist from the same hospital that diagnosed me. Which happened to be the same hospital that the woman sharing the story was employed by. She disclosed that her sister was diagnosed with cancer in her genitals. Initially, her sister was present for chemotherapy, but after a while, the woman received a call as her emergency contact. Her sister had not been attending treatment for weeks. She asked her sister why she was not going to treatment and she informed her that the diagnosis, as well as the treatment process, hurt unbearably. She urged her sister to take the process of treating this "monster" seriously, but her words were to no avail. Her sister succumbed to cancer nine months after her initial diagnosis. She was only 58 years old. My husband and I were speechless! I instantly thought about my grandfather and aunt who had also died from cancer. Actually, I witnessed my aunt wither away from cancer in her early forties. I could not imagine leaving my family behind for any reason, let alone for something as mysterious as cancer. The woman went on to ask us what our plans were and who we were consulting. We informed her that we were told by MSK that we would have to provide them with ALL of my medical records before being seen. Even though we had access to the patient portal like everyone else, I did not know what specific records they needed or where I would go to print this obviously large amount of paperwork. The woman looked at me and my husband for a second or less and offered to print out my records. This printing process took her about 15 minutes. When it was all said and done, she had printed out over 100 pages of medical records. Finally, we were beginning to see some form of good fortune from this nightmare. Before we got up to leave, my husband asked her if she thought it would be wise for us to stick with the doctor that diagnosed me, be willing to begin treatment immediately, or should we be patient with MSK, submit the documentation, and allow them to treat me. Without hesitation, she informed us that if her sister had been treated or consulted MSK for that matter, she would be alive today. We could not thank her enough for all she had done for us. It was like GOD whispered in her ears and she granted HIS wishes without a second thought. Truly, this encounter felt like "fate".

The very next day, we informed the kind woman that my husband spoke to a few days ago regarding our set of circumstances that we had the materials requested. She informed us that we could bring the slides to MSK, but we would have to email the documents straight to her because she was working from home due to the pandemic and needed to put my records in the system for the doctors' review. Without the records, the oncologist would dare not to look at the slides. We reached out to the guy that is always there to "save the day" as his entire family's knight in shining armor. My husband's father took the documents to his office, which was closed due to COVID, and contacted one of its office managers. Although she had been working from home for the past 6 months, she came all the way from Long Island into the city, scanned and emailed all 100 plus pieces of my records. After a few days of patiently waiting for some sort of contact from MSK, we received the call that we could come in for a consultation to discuss my situation. On that day, we encountered a breath of fresh air that would shed light on this extremely grim turn of events. She would serve as my oncologist throughout my road to recovery. My husband and I awaited her entry into the examination room, not knowing if we would get the same sort of feedback we received when I was initially diagnosed. She walked in with a bright smile as though we were there for a routine physical. She asked me how I was feeling and proceeded to examine my breast. My husband immediately interrupted the exam and asked if she read through the records and viewed the scans. She assured him that she had. Then, the answer to his next question I would say served as the turning point of my outlook on this ordeal. He informed her that the diagnosing doctor told us that she had four to five years to live at best. Then he asked her what her take was. With a calm, cool, collected tone, she replied, "We do not give our patients expiration dates here." My husband and I looked at one another with the longest sigh of relief. Even though she was not GOD, at that point we truly believed that this place along with our faith would repair my internal wounds. After the examination, I was introduced to another delightful young woman who would serve as my nurse during this time. She gave me her cellular number and encouraged me to call at any time should I be experiencing any pain or to simply get things off my chest. After a few hours at MSK, we felt like we were summoned here by GOD and that we were truly in good hands.

The night before my chemotherapy had finally arrived. At this point, I had waist-length hair and had witnessed how my family members who were diagnosed with cancer shed every strand of hair on their bodies. I decided to not allow this disease to control this facet of my appearance. Therefore, me and my eight-year-old daughter cut, snipped and devoured every inch of my hair that I used to cherish as something that made a woman, a woman. By midnight, I was completely bald and truly felt free from fear of the unknown as well as having to wash my hair every few days. I was scheduled for chemotherapy once a week and would be given a single medication for chemo and 2 antibody medications during my 3-hour treatments. Obviously, I was oblivious to the side effects of any of these federally allocated drugs. I expected a reaction, but nothing as adverse as what I encountered. Before every treatment, the patient must draw a few vials of blood to ensure there are not any impurities that would interfere with the treatment process. After waiting for about an hour of being cleared for treatment, I was escorted to my own room with a leather recliner and flat-screen television. I was informed by the nurse that I would have both hands and feet placed in ice to slow down the deterioration of my nails. Within another 30 minutes, it was time to receive my very first chemotherapy. I was then told that I would be given a medication named *Taxol*. A needle was poked in my chest, basically implanted in the port I was given a month and a half prior to this experience. On my left side, sat the intravenous (IV) with the medication that I would later learn was of a generic sort. After about 40 seconds of therapy, my entire body went numb, and my chest felt as though a 300-pound boulder was placed on top of it. I could not breathe. During initial treatments, a nurse stays in the room with the patient on guard for incidents like this. Originally, I thought this was my body getting used to an unknown substance. However, when I could not move my facial muscles and asked the nurse was, I was supposed to feel this way, I knew something was terribly wrong. She summoned other nurses and the physician. They immediately unhooked me from the (IV) and replaced it with Benadryl. After being asked if I could move my limbs and make a smile, which I could do neither, I blacked out for roughly 4 hours. When I awoke, I was informed that they notified my husband who was obviously frantic but was assured that he had nothing to worry about. My father-in-law and husband picked me up from MSK and I could not truly explain why this had occurred. The very next day, my oncologist called me, providing the information that changed my outlook on

184

the business of "treating" ailments in America. As noted, I was given the generic form of *Taxol*. After speaking with the oncologist and then doing my own research, I revealed that there is a higher quality of *Taxol* that an insurance company will not cover UNLESS a life-threatening occurrence takes place such as mine. Therefore, if the generic drug does not kill you, then they will continue to treat a patient with it. I have encountered a few women that have been on chemotherapy for years and ironically enough are still being treated with the lower-level product. These very women are withering away in front of their physicians' eyes. My oncologist informed me that I would be scheduled for the following week but will be treated with the higher quality form of *Taxol*. Basically, MSK had them provide the insurance company with substantial proof that I almost died due to the ill-advised reaction to the generic drug.

When that day came to receive the higher-quality treatment, I was still apprehensive. Because at this point, it seemed as though my life was practically in the insurance company's hands. I came in, did the routine blood work, was approved for treatment after about an hour, and was seated in the same room I blacked out in. The nurse poked me in the chest with the needle and continued to hook me up to the IV. The ice packs were placed on my limbs. Then, I sat there waiting—expecting the worst. So, I waited, waited, and waited. And nothing happened! Only a cold tingly sensation went through my body as if it was being rejuvenated. An hour later, I was given the 2 antibody treatments that would hopefully protect my organs from being infected with cancer as they were being healed by the chemotherapy. After an hour and a half of this treatment, I was mentally, emotionally, and physically exhausted. When I got home, all I did was sleep for hours. Thank GOD I have the resources of my family to tend to the needs of my children during this phase in my life. My heart truly goes out to people that do not have the support of anyone while facing the challenge of not being able to physically do what they normally do or mentally muster up the energy to think about anything past their upcoming treatment.

For the next three to four months of weekly treatment, I experienced daily headaches, body aches, abrupt mood swings, and endless diarrhea. It was hard to keep in mind that I was enduring all this discomfort en route to possibly ridding myself of cancer. I would see my oncologist every other week to keep her abreast of how I felt as far as the toll the treatment was having on my wellbeing. She encouraged me to see a therapist to which I was referred to that was well versed in treating those with cancer diagnoses. I was a bit hesitant because I had never sat and spoken to a stranger about myself, but at this point, it could not hurt after all I had been through. After a few sessions, it was clear that I would have benefited more from someone that could truly identify with how I was feeling, as a woman. My mental health therapeutic experience was not bad at all, but I would say it is imperative for those diagnosed with cancer to seek mental health therapy (as everyone should) and be proactive in selecting someone that meets your personal criteria(s).

My oncologist informed me that I would have to get a full-body scan to determine if cancer had traveled to other parts of my body and how well the treatment was working, if at all. Once again, I did not know what to expect. I had only been on chemotherapy for four months, so what were the chances that it worked in such a short period of time. I had the pet scan, which I had become accustomed to receiving, and I was told that the doctor would complete a phone visit on Monday morning. Ironically enough, Monday was the 16th anniversary of the day my husband and I met. We woke up bright and early, took the phone off silent, and awaited the news that could once again change our lives forever. At 11 am, promptly, she called with her usual vibrant demeanor, initially asking us how we were doing. We informed her that today was a special day for us, and she noted that she would relay the news that would make it even better. The scans showed that I had no sign of cancer and that all 10 lesions had disintegrated. We were speechless! As we both smiled ear to ear like the Grinch, all we both could do is cry and sob in happiness. But what did this really mean for us moving forward? She informed me that I would be taken off chemotherapy and would begin to receive only antibody treatment weekly for the next month or so. Thereafter, I would receive antibody medication every three weeks, probably for the rest of my life, to protect my body from developing cancer in the future. After being taken off chemotherapy, I could feel my body beginning to get stronger and life was beginning to go back to normal. After my three-week antibody treatment began, my husband asked me if we should resume our plans to move south again. We both agreed that the past nine months had certainly tested our faith in our HIGHER POWER and that it was now time to move forward with our lives. During the summer, my husband landed the federal job that he had been applying for a few years. Also, I located a local cancer center in the south to take the helm of administering my antibody treatments. My girls were enrolled into a good school nearby the very home in the south I sit in today while writing this memoir. And after three trimester CT scans, I am free of fear, free of pain, and by the grace of GOD, free of cancer.

Scriptures For Healing

Hosea 4:6
My people are destroyed for lack of knowledge.

Galatians 3:13
Christ has redeemed us from the curse of the law, having become a curse for us...

1 Peter 2:24
(Jesus) bore our sins in His own body on the tree, that we, having died to sins, might live for righteousness -- by whose stripes you were healed.

Isaiah 53:5
He was wounded for our transgressions, He was bruised for our iniquities; the chastisement for our peace was upon Him, and by His stripes we are healed.

Matthew 8:17
He Himself took our infirmities and bore our sicknesses.

Psalm 107:20
He sent His word and healed them, and delivered them from their destructions.

Proverbs 3:7
Do not be wise in your own eyes: fear the Lord and depart from evil.

Proverbs 3:8
It will be health to your flesh, and strength to your bones.

Exodus 15:26
I am the Lord who heals you.

Psalm 103:3
Who forgives all your iniquities, Who heals all your diseases.

Exodus 23:25
And ye shall serve the Lord your God, and He will bless your bread and your water. And I will take sickness away from the midst of you.

Proverbs 16:24
Pleasant words are like a honeycomb, sweetness to the soul and hearth to the bones.

Isaiah 58:8
Your light shall break forth like the morning, your healing shall spring forth speedily, and your righteousness shall go before you; the glory of the Lord shall be your rear guard.

Psalm 118:17
I shall not die, but live, and declare the works of the Lord.

Psalm 147:3
He heals the brokenhearted and binds up their wounds.

Proverbs 17:22
A merry heart does good, like a medicine, but a broken spirit dries the bones.

3 John 2
Beloved, I pray that you may prosper in all things and be in health, just as your soul prospers.

Mark 16:17
These signs will follow those who believe: In My name they will cast out demons; they will speak with new tongues; ...they will lay hands on the sick, and they will recover.

James 5:15
The prayer of faith will save the sick, and the Lord will raise him up. And if he has committed sins, he will be forgiven.

James 5:16
Confess your trespasses to one another, and pray for one another, that you may be healed.

Reflection Journal
It's Your Turn

"A Shoe has so much more to offer than just a walk"
Author Unknown

This collection of writings was designed to empower and motivate you. View this body of writing as a toolkit, how might you proceed on your personal journey. Below you will find reflection questions that will aide in your initial steps in drafting you own story; for pure reflection, for encouraging another, or to simply tell your story. Just as we took up this responsibility in designing this book to provide hope for someone else, we hold you accountable to continue the journey. **It's your turn!**

1. How has your life changed since breast cancer?

2. What does your support system look like or where did you find it?

3. What advice would you give to yourself?

4. What are some words of hope and advice that you would share with someone who is being impacted by breast cancer?

Dear BREASTie...This Is My Story

Meet The Co-Authors

Tamekia Hunter Ross

Tamekia Hunter Ross a/k/a *"Minister T"*, is a proud 1992 graduate of Sumter High School and thereafter received a Bachelor of Science Degree in Political Science/Pre-Law from Francis Marion University in 1996. She has over twenty-five years of experience as a Paralegal in various types of law with a primary focus in Bankruptcy Law. After spending twenty years as a Paralegal, *"Minister T"* accepted a career transition in 2017 and currently works at Burnette Shutt & McDaniel Law Firm as their Intake Process Manager in Columbia, South Carolina. In November 2014, *"Minister T"* graduated from the Sonship School of the First Born under the leadership of the Late Bishop Nate Holcombe and The Christian House of Prayer (Killeen, Texas). Thereafter, she received a Certificate of License and Ordination in February 2015. She serves as one of the Associate Ministers of Victory Church. In her spare time, you may find her shopping for shoes, handbags, and accessories that were captivated by her former Glam boutique business in Greenville, South Carolina. She is a living testament of God's grace, mercy, and power within us. She travels every three weeks to the Cancer Treatment Centers in Newnan, Georgia for ongoing chemotherapy treatment for Stage IV Metastatic Breast Cancer. While battling and fighting for her life daily, God gives her the strength to get through 12-hour days of commuting and work and coming home to be a full-time wife and mother. You will often hear her say, "I don't look like what I am going through". She is a native and current resident of Sumter, South Carolina. She is all smiles when it comes to being a devoted wife to the "Love of her Life" Arnteyus "A.J." Ross, and mother to her boys, Cameron and Caleb. Together they have a blended family of six children and a bonus grandson who calls her "GLAM-Ma". Minister T lives life daily giving God back His word, "Daughter (Tamekia), your Faith has healed you from Stage IV Metastatic Breast Cancer. Go in peace and be free of your infirmities". On her bad days, she reminds herself of what God promised her, "This sickness (Metastatic Breast Cancer) will not end in death but so the son of God, Jesus Christ, will be glorified." Breast Cancer is just a platform Minister T uses to give Him Glory and draw people closer to Jesus because we were created to be Faith Strong!

Angela S. Ashley

I am Angela S. Ashley, born September 19, 1955, in Gastonia, N.C. I am married to Rev. Charles L. Ashley, Sr.; we reside in Gastonia, North Carolina. We are the parents of Litisha D. Ashley and Charles L. Ashley, Jr. I prefer Psalms 23 as my favorite scripture because, during my ordeal as a two-time cancer survivor, this passage gave me strength and courage to continue trusting and believing that God is my shepherd, and I shall not want. I maintained my faith and confidence that God would heal me. After graduating from Hunter Huss High, Gastonia, N.C., I chose Early Childhood Education as my field of endeavor; I attended Gaston College, Dallas N.C., where I received certification to teach Head Start. My favorite and fun things I enjoy are home interior decorating, cooking, exercising, and listening to music. Some of my fun facts are having a sense of humor and a willingness to laugh; because laughter is the best medicine, it is good for the soul. I have served as the First Lady of Galilee Baptist Church, York, South Carolina, for 25 years.

Dr. Bernice H. Mullins

Dr. Bernice H. Mullins is the 10th child of the late Stephen Marion and Mary D. Heyward of Sumter South Carolina. She was the wife of the late Bishop Roger W. Mullins. She has three children, Renata, Roger JT, and Ricardo. She is blessed to have 6 grandchildren. There are so many children that claim her as a mom that were once her students in the educational system. She has recently retired from being an educator/administrator with 43 years in education. She received her BA in Elementary Education, Masters in Education, Education Specialist in Education, Doctorate Degree in Christian Education and Ministry, and is a certified Grief Counselor. She is a member of Bible Outreach Ministries COGIC where Elder Calvin E. Peterson is Pastor and Auxiliary Bishop Keith Kershaw is the Superintendent, and Bishop William A. Prioleau, Presiding Prelate of the state of South Carolina. She is a Bible Band teacher and is the supervisor of the Evangelism Department. She is also a member of Delta Sigma Theta Sorority Inc. She is a published author of a Children's book, I Can't Wait Until Morning, and her latest book, Mercy for the Bereaved; A Journey Through the Death of a Soulmate, which she wrote as she battled cancer while on chemotherapy. These books are available through most book outlets. Dr. Mullins states that she is determined to share her testimony and to share the gospel of Jesus Christ every chance that she gets. She wants everyone to remember that "If God allows you to be in a trial, He has the power to bring you through it. Whatever the outcome, we win because we belong to God." We're "UNSTOPPABLE" (Koryn Hawthorne, Gospel Artist.).

Bertha L. Johnson

Bertha Johnson is currently a Section Chief, Information Services Unit at the Department of Homeland Security (DHS), U.S. Citizenship and Immigration Services (USCIS), Houston Field Office. Since August 25, 2013, Ms. Johnson has served in the Houston Field Office, Houston, Texas as a Section Chief whose portfolios have included the Adjustment of Status, Information Services, and Records Management Programs, Congressional, and Application Support Centers. Prior to entering on duty at the Houston Field Office, she had over 16 years of experience working in the contracting field administering multi-million-dollar contracts for multiple locations with legacy INS and the Department of Homeland Security. Bertha is a native of South Carolina and attended Cortez Peters Business College in Washington, D. C. and has completed many college credit hour courses and career developmental courses. Through continuing education, she earned an Associate's and a Master's Certificate in Project Management. She is divorced and has one son, Gilbert, and a daughter-in-law, Danielle.

Chelia "Lia" Frank

Chelia "Lia" Frank was born in Secaucus, New Jersey, and raised in Irvington for 16 years. She is the daughter of Levan and Millie Frank and the youngest of five siblings. She began her education in Essex County until the end of 2000. Her family then moved to Clarendon County, and she graduated with honors from Scott's Branch High in 2002. She then went on to obtain her Associate's degree in Science and a certificate in Pharmacy Tech from Columbia College, of Columbia, South Carolina, and a certificate of completion for medical billing and coding from Ultimate Medical Academy. Along with certifications in phlebotomy, EKG, and certified nursing assistant from Allheart in Sumter, South Carolina. She is engaged to Willie McCray Jr and mother of two wonderful girls, Toni and Taylor, along with six bonus children. She currently resides in Sumter, South Carolina, where she currently receives her treatments between Prisma Health Tuomey Cancer Treatment Center of Sumter and South Carolina Oncology, of Columbia, South Carolina. Her love for helping and caring for others has kept her working in the medical field at Sumter Pediatrics for over 5 years. She enjoys traveling, riding motorcycles with her fiancé, and has a passion for trying new DIY projects with her children. She is a member of her family church at Greater St. Phillip RUME of Pinewood, South Carolina along with often visiting Mt. Nebo Baptist Church in Alcolu, South Carolina. In May of 2021, at the age of 37, she was diagnosed with Stage 2 invasive ductal carcinoma, which forever changed her life.

Harriett D. Reynolds

Harriett D. Brown-Reynolds is the Founder of Financial Independence Starts Here (F.I.S.H); a division of HVB Enterprises, LLC. She is also a certified Financial Health Coach. Her purpose and passion are focused on supporting individuals on their road to financial independence and to enjoy life. Harriett's professional experience includes over 13 years in the banking industry. Harriett has also served over 15 years in the non-profit sector as Chief Program Officer, Financial Stability Program Manager, Credit Counselor, Housing Counselor, and currently as the Financial Empowerment Lead at an agency whose mission is to house homeless families. Harriett's utmost source of inspiration came from her mom, Helen Virginia Brown (HVB), her relationship with the Lord and the love of her family. Harriett is dedicated to serving others and finds her greatest joy when she can help change lives. Harriett lives in Knightdale, NC and has one adult son, Steven A. Reynolds.

Jennyveia K. Persaud

Jennyveia K. Persaud is a native of Guyana, South America. Ms. Peraud grew up as an only child, which triggered her individuality, imagination, and integrity. Her hobbies include ANYTHING that encourages creativity, free-thinking, and a passion for prosperity. Ms. Persaud is a licensed Cosmetologist and owner of *Jennyveia's Beauty salon.* Jennyviea is married to her childhood sweetheart, LaQuon, and a mother of two girls, Ava-Monet and Eva-Monae.

Karen Owens Blanding

Karen was born at Shaw, Air Force Base, and has lived in Sumter, South Carolina all of her life. She is the daughter of Wilhelmenia Owens and the late Tony Owens, Jr., and the baby sister of Antonio "Squeaky" Owens. Bernard Blanding is her phenomenal husband and they have three sons. MiSTER Cornelius Blanding, Cordell Blanding, and Camron Blanding. Karen graduated from Sumter High School in 1981 and furthered her education at South Carolina State University by earning a B.A and M.A. in Speech Pathology and Audiology, 1985 and 1991 respectively. She has been a licensed Speech-Language Pathologist since 1991. She became a proud member of Alpha Kappa Alpha Sorority, Inc. Spring of 1982, Beta Sigma Chapter at South Carolina State University, and is currently a life member. Karen worships at St. Mark Four Bridges Missionary Baptist Church, Sumter, South Carolina, under the leadership of Pastor Sammie D. Simmons, where they are taught to walk in their ordained destiny. She has created www.karenblanding.com to provide information and strategies to early interventionist and caregivers in hopes of helping infants and toddlers develop early developmental skills. She also has a passion for baking homemade fruitcakes that taste like your great grandmother made them. Learn more about them by visiting www.fruitcakebykaren.com. and she has recently added the skill of crocheting hats and scarves as a hobby to help with the cost of medical expenses. Visit www.crochetbykaren.com to make a donation to support.

Kathy N. Bellamy

Kathy Bellamy is the daughter of the late Charlie and Margaret Nelson. She is a 1984 graduate of Manning High School. She graduated from Morris College, Sumter, South Carolina, with a Bachelor of Science Degree in Business Management. She is a member of Mt. Chapel Baptist Church, Manning, South Carolina, where she's active in various ministries. She is a member of the illustrious Delta Sigma Theta Sorority, Inc, and is active in the Sumter Alumnae Chapter, Sumter, South Carolina. Kathy is married to her husband, Mark of 31 years. Kathy loves people and believes in treating others the way she wants to be treated. Reading is her favorite pastime. She is a breast cancer survivor who wants to share hope with others. She is Faith Strong.

Kelli McNeill-Wilhelm

Kelli is a North Carolina native and currently resides in the Raleigh/Durham area with her husband, Wayne. They are the parents of four young adults, Nikki, Jordan, Jada and Justin, and the proud Grandparents (Ahma and Papa) to four exceptionally perfect grandchildren, Aubriyauna, Milyn, Rylee and Omari. She received her Bachelor of Arts in Psychology from the University of North Carolina, Chapel Hill. She works full time within the Child Welfare field in local government. Kelli's most rewarding (and sometimes challenging) job is being yoked together in Pastoral ministry with her husband—mostly providing an outlet for him to vent, brainstorm, and share ideas and revelations as he leads a small but impactful congregation in Durham, NC. In her spare time, she enjoys traveling with her husband, binge watching TV shows on various streaming outlets, and relaxing on her back deck with a good book. She draws an exorbitant amount of energy from and has a passion for, advocating for marginalized communities, groups, and people. She is a first-time author.

Kimberly S. Curtis

Kimberly S. Curtis, a native Washingtonian, a child of the Most High God, a blessed wife, a proud Mother of two, and the grateful grandmother of three. I earned my ASN at Prince George's Community College and my BSN at the University of Phoenix. I am a Pediatric Registered Nurse at Children's Hospital in Washington, DC. I am also an entrepreneur (baker) of Kakes By Kim LLC. I enjoy baking, bowling, traveling, spending time with my family, and serving the community. I am a member of the Life After Cancer Ministry at Faith United Ministries and an active member of Chi Eta Phi Sorority, Inc. Alpha Chapter. I know I have been called to serve. I pray I can encourage someone as I strive daily to live for Jesus. One of my favorite scripture references is Philippians 4:13.

Kimberly W. Herrington

Kimberly W. Herrington is a Permanency Manager with Wake County Health & Human Services. She is a native of Chicago, Illinois, and began her career as a Social Worker with the Illinois Department of Children & Family Services. She transitioned to Raleigh, North Carolina over 25 years ago. Kimberly has dedicated her career to Child Welfare Services for over 30 years. In her current role, she serves as the manager for Foster Parent Recruitment; Licensing; Adoption/Post Adoption Services; Kinship Licensure; Guardianship Assistance Program; and Foster Care Medicaid Eligibility. In other positions, Kimberly has served as a Permanency Services Social Worker, LINKS Social Worker, and Adolescent Foster Care Supervisor. Kimberly has dedicated her career to serving children and building the capacity of families adding timely permanency and improved well-being for children. She has also been a strong advocate for parents and building strong communities. When she is not making magic happen, she enjoys spending time at the beach, reading a book, or gardening. She earned a Bachelor of Arts degree in Psychology from Western Illinois University and a Master of Arts degree in Psychology from Chicago State University.

Linda Mahoney

Linda Mahoney is the epitome of a Virtuous Woman. She is the mother of one son. She is a graduate of Hillcrest High School. She earned her Bachelor of Business Administration from Allen University. She is an Accountant in the Medical field. She enjoys worshiping God, traveling, dancing, singing, walking, meeting people, and spending time with family, especially her son. She is a proud member of Alpha Kappa Alpha Sorority, Inc. Her favorite scripture is Psalms 121.

Linda Tyrice Jefferson

Linda Tyrice Jefferson was born in Washington, DC, and is the oldest daughter of the late Theresa Jefferson. She is also the eldest granddaughter of Annie Mahoney. She has three wonderful children. One son, John Jefferson and two daughters Samaria & Sierra Holton. She is a new and proud grandma of two grandsons. She lives her life with the "Serenity Prayer". She works as a Surgical Ophthalmologist Technician at Med Star Georgetown Hospital is affiliated with Med Star Franklin Square Hospital She has also worked as a Licensed Practical Nurse. She is a 1989 graduate of Bladensburg High School, 1992 and a graduate of Germanna Community College School of Nursing, and a 2011 Graduate of the Dulaney Eye Institute. She is a long time member at Victory Grace Church in Bladensburg, MD under the biblical teaching of Dr. Jasmine"Jazz" Sculark. In her spare time, she loves Black history, hiking, learning from the seniors, and dancing. She also enjoys laughing and spending time with her family. Nature is her first love. She finds joy in nature. This is the place where she can find and spend time with God.

MaryAnn Williams

MaryAnn Peterson Williams is the oldest child of the late Alex and Gladys Mahoney Peterson. Her maternal family, James, Sr and Katie Wactor Jenkins Mahoney, reared her. She is the second oldest of seven children in this blended family. She is from Sumter, S.C. She is the mother of one child, Ramsey Williams. She has spent 25 years working in the telecommunications and customer service industry. Ms. Williams has spent the last 14 years in public service working for the United States Senate, as a call center manager. She has earned her BA in Human Resources from Strayer University, Master of Administration, in Human Resources from Central Michigan University. She also has a Master of Science in IT Project Management, from George Washington University. She gained a great deal of her biblical understanding from her early years at Mt. Olive AME Church. She is active in her workplace Bible Study, under the teachings of Dr. Barry Black. She attends Metropolitan Baptist Church in Largo, MD, she studies under the teaching of Dr. Maurice Watson. MaryAnn enjoys time with family and friends. She often states that it is so fortunate to have friends that have become family. In her spare time, she enjoys traveling, fine dining, and creating. She has her own crafting business, specializing in unique gift baskets.

Michele A. Washington

Michele A. Washington hails from Lynn, Massachusetts. She is the second of six children born to the late Robert Pedro and the late Joan Lambertis Pedro. She currently resides in South Carolina. She is married and has a son, a daughter, and four grandchildren. She is a retired Combat Veteran from the Air Forces Reserves. She served a combined total of 26 years in the Air Force (including active duty) and the Navy Reserves. During the first half of her Military career, she was a Jet Engine Mechanic, later changing to an Air Transportation Specialist. Currently retired, she devotes her time to her church, family, her dogs, volunteering with various agencies, and traveling.

Jean Bailey

I was born on August 11, 1937, to William and Mable Evans. At the time of my birth, African-American women did not give birth in hospitals, so I was born, with the assistance of a midwife on Wade Avenue in Raleigh, NC. I have grown up in Raleigh all my life and graduated from J. W. Ligon High School in 1955. My class was the second graduating class from Ligon, as it was built in 1953 as the all-black high school in the city of Raleigh. I loved my time in high school, and was the lead majorette for J. W. Ligon. This is also where I met my first husband and the father of my four children. My husband and I raised our two daughters and two sons together but later divorced in 1976. I was fortunate to have a career as an accounting clerk at D. H. Hill Library on the campus of North Carolina State University. I retired from that career in 1997.

Stacey Haywood

Stacey Haywood, an ordained Elder in the Mount Calvary Holy Church of America, currently serving locally in Mount Calvary Word of Faith, Raleigh, NC. I am the honored wife of Theodore Haywood, and the proud mother of two adult children Shamella McDaniel, and Jahiem Haywood. I currently hold a BS

Degree in Religion, from the University of Mount Olive. I am the founder and CEO of What's Underneath Matters, LLC, a non-profit organization that provides undergarments to low-income, at-risk youth with a scope on those in the foster care system in Wake County and surrounding areas. I am a full-time Insurance Adjuster, licensed in over 28 states. I am eternally grateful to The Lord for restoration and the ability to wear many hats and still live my life on purpose to the fullest.

Tamara Wactor

Tamara Wactor is a native of Sumter, South Carolina. She is a 1996 graduate of Hillcrest High School. She is a member of Mt. Olive AME Church in Woodrow, South Carolina. She is active in the Women's Missionary Society and a member of the J & I Mass Choir. Tamara enjoys singing in the choir, spending time with her family and friends, social events, and enjoying life. As she evolves in her life's goals, she continues to uplift others in their journey. She believes in keeping God first. Her greatest joy is spending time with her two children.

Tammey Davis

Tammey Davis is a native of Hopkins, South Carolina. She is a Lower Richland graduate along with a graduate of Morris College of Sumter where she obtained a Bachelor's degree in Science going to Limestone to receive a Master's in Criminology. She is the mother of two sons, Landen and Cassius Bannister. She is the youngest of three girls. She is a member of Zion Benevolent Baptist church and a member of the Order of Eastern Star and Zeta Phi Beta Sorority Inc. Tammy is also a Columbia Fire department honor guard. She served in the United States Army for 20 years. She is a member of the Wounded Warrior Project. She has a passion for living life.

Tomika L. Marks

My name is Tomika L. Marks. I have been married to my husband, Justin for 20 years. We have two beautiful children, Kennedi, who is 16, and Peyton, who is 14. I am originally from Sumter, South Carolina, and a graduate of Hillcrest High School in '96. I live in Nashville, TN, and have been here for the past 13 years. I am currently a program coordinator at Vanderbilt University Medical Center.

Willene Thomasena Wactor Brisbone

First and foremost, Willene Thomasena Wactor Brisbone is a child of the "most-high" God and at a very early age dedicated her life to serving Him. One of Willene's favorite scriptures is Philippians 4:13, "I can do all things through Christ which strengthens me". Willene was born in Sumter County, South Carolina, and is the oldest child (out of seven) of Thomas and Rosa Elizabeth Wilson Wactor, both deceased. Willene is a very active member of Mt. Olive

African Methodist Episcopal (AME) Church in Woodrow, South Carolina, where she serves as a Steward, a Class Leader, a member of the Women Missionary Society, member of the Senior Unity Choir, member of the Praise & Worship Team, member of the Church School (aka Sunday School), member of the Stewardess Board, member of the Lay Organization, and participates in Bible Study and other church ministries such as Captain of the church Sumter County American Cancer Society Relay for Life Team. Willene married Albert Brisbone, Sr. on February 20, 1967. They were married for over 50 years until Albert's death on June 30, 2017. From this union, they had four beautiful children (Albert Jr-deceased, Lisa, Randy, and Marcus), a daughter-in-law (Renesha), seven grandchildren (Shericka, Randy Jr, Jennifer, Nylisha, Ramikis, Jayce, and Jana), and four great-grands (Iris, Kennedy, Azalea, Zuri).

We Are Faith Strong

Inviting all Breast Cancer Survivors, Thrivers and Metavivors to join the Faith Strong Support Group!

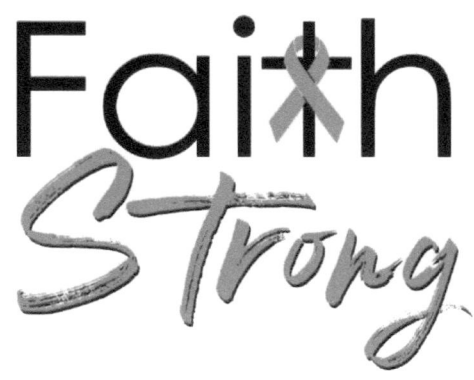

The mission of Faith Strong is to provide relational, emotional, and spiritual support to breast cancer Thrivers, Survivors, and Metaviors while advocating and educating our community about breast cancer.

We BELIEVE
But He was wounded for our transgressions, He was bruised for our iniquities: the chastisement of our peace was upon Him; and with His stripes we are **HEALED.**
Isaiah 53:5

Contact Us:
info@wearefaithstrong.com

www.wearefaithstrong.com

PO BOX 3398
Sumter, SC 29151